Artificial Intelligence in Dentistry

Khalid Shaikh • Sreelekshmi Vivek Bekal
Hesham Fathi Ahmed Marei
Walid Shaaban Moustafa Elsayed
Dusan Surdilovic • Lubna Abdel Jawad

Artificial Intelligence in Dentistry

Springer

Khalid Shaikh
Prognica Labs Tech FZCO
Dubai, United Arab Emirates

Sreelekshmi Vivek Bekal
IntelliDent AI
Dubai, United Arab Emirates

Hesham Fathi Ahmed Marei
Gulf Medical University
Ajman, United Arab Emirates

Walid Shaaban Moustafa Elsayed
Gulf Medical University
Ajman, United Arab Emirates

Dusan Surdilovic
Gulf Medical University
Ajman, United Arab Emirates

Lubna Abdel Jawad
Gulf Medical University
Ajman, United Arab Emirates

ISBN 978-3-031-19714-7 ISBN 978-3-031-19715-4 (eBook)
https://doi.org/10.1007/978-3-031-19715-4

This Springer imprint is published by the registered company Springer Nature Switzerland AG
The registered company address is: Gewerbestrasse 11, 6330 Cham, Switzerland

Preface

Dentistry is one of the earliest specialties of medicine, dating back to 7000 BCE. Over time, dentistry and dental care blazed the trail to evolve from a primitive form of medicine to its present-day iteration of preventative dental care, state-of-the-art diagnostics, and modern-age treatment. From theories of dental diseases caused by "evil spirits" and "tooth worms" to the latest cutting-edge technologies using artificial intelligence, dentistry has come a long way! Despite all these advancements, less work is done in this area of specialization when it comes to knowledge and skills in medical science and engineering background for diagnosis and further maintenance of oral health.

Our book carefully articulates all aspects of dentistry, compiling the history, anatomy, and specialties of dentistry, most significant dental health conditions and their implications on global health, current technological advancements, and potential areas of artificial intelligence applications in this domain. This research work is a culmination of engineering skills and medical background in an area of great interest to the medical community. By sincerely contributing to this research work for technological evolution, we strongly advocate for the FDI World Dental Federation's report.

Vision 2030: Delivering Optimal Oral Health for All. Finally, deep learning AI models, including their performance within the classification of dental diseases, are introduced and detailed in our effort.

We sincerely hope that we can contribute to the eventual technological evolution within the early detection of cancer.

Overview of the Book

In Chap. 1, basic information on dentistry and its history, evolution, and specialties, are discussed. The basics of dental anatomy, nomenclature, and developmental disturbances are finely discussed in Chap. 2. Significant oral health conditions are described in Chap. 3, followed by a careful deliberation of the impact of oral health on global health in Chap. 4. In Chap. 5, advancements in dentistry are mentioned. Information on artificial intelligence and various learning algorithms are covered in Chap. 6, including the working of various learning algorithm's advantages and limitations. Chapter 7 focuses on the impact of AI on global health, followed by the applications of AI in oral health and imaging. Machine learning in dentistry is covered in Chap. 8, where it meticulously describes how AI assists in teeth identification and caries detection, alongside cavity detection, using deep learning.

Features of the Book

- Basic information on dentistry and oral health
- Dental anatomy, tooth notation, and nomenclature
- Most common oral diseases
- Impact of oral health on global health
- Advancements in dentistry
- Details of learning algorithms and their role in healthcare and dental imaging
- Computer-aided system for detection of oral health conditions
- Inclusion of deep learning model for detection and diagnosis of caries

Acknowledgments

My task has been easier and the final version of the book considerably better because of the help we have received. I would also like to thank the publishers at Springer, in particular Michael McCabe, Senior Editor, and Arjun Narayan, Project Coordinator, for their helpful guidance and encouragement during the creation of this book.

Dubai, UAE Khalid Shaikh
Dubai, UAE Sreelekshmi Vivek Bekal
Ajman, UAE Hesham Fathi Ahmed Marei
Ajman, UAE Walid Shaaban Moustafa Elsayed
Ajman, UAE Dusan Surdilovic
Ajman, UAE Lubna Abdel Jawad

Contents

Chapter 1
Introduction to Dentistry and Oral Health

1.1 What Is Dentistry?

1.1.1 Definition of Dentistry

Dentistry is defined as the evaluation, diagnosis, prevention, and/or treatment (non-surgical, surgical, or related procedures) of diseases, disorders, and/or conditions of the oral cavity, maxillofacial area, and/or the adjacent and associated structures and their impact on the human body, provided by a dentist, within the scope of his/her education, training, and experience, in accordance with the ethics of the profession and applicable law (Adopted, American Dental Association House of Delegates, 10/21/97) [1].

Dentistry is also defined as the profession concerned with the prevention and treatment of oral disease, including diseases of the teeth, and supporting structures and diseases of the soft tissues of the mouth. It also encompasses the treatment and correction of malformation of the jaws, misalignment of the teeth, and birth anomalies of the oral cavity such as cleft palate. In addition to general practice, dentistry includes many specialties and subspecialties, including orthodontics and dental orthopedics, pediatric dentistry, periodontics, prosthodontics, oral and maxillofacial surgery, oral and maxillofacial pathology, endodontics, public health dentistry, and oral and maxillofacial radiology [2].

Dentistry is often also understood to subsume the now largely defunct medical specialty of stomatology (the study of the mouth and its disorders and diseases) for which reason the two terms are used interchangeably in certain regions [3] (Fig. 1.1).

Dentistry is thought to have been the first specialization in medicine which has gone on to develop its own accredited degree with its own specializations. The current approach of evidence-based dentistry judiciously integrates the dentist's clinical expertise, the patient's need and preferences, and the most current, clinically relevant evidence to lead in the promotion of oral health by disseminating the best

K. Shaikh et al., *Artificial Intelligence in Dentistry*,
https://doi.org/10.1007/978-3-031-19715-4_1

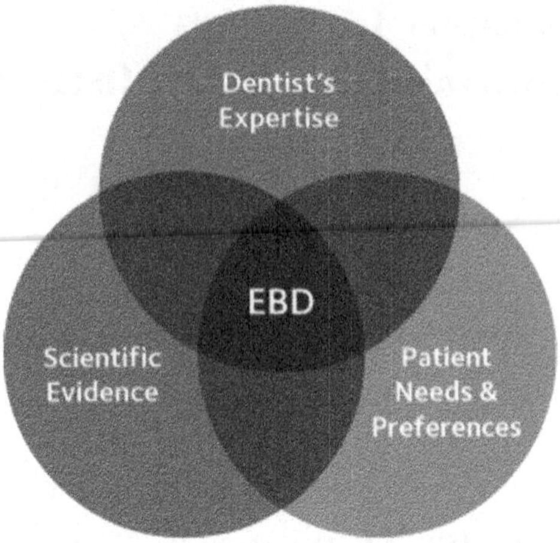

Fig. 1.1 Evidence-based dentistry

available scientific information and helping practitioners implement it into clinical practice, thereby improving their decision-making and standard of care.

Evidence-based dentistry is also implemented in radiology to aid in diagnosis and treatment and hematology (study of blood), to provide robust scientific evidence, and to enhance this clinical protocol, cardiology (due to various severe complications arising from dental surgery in patients with heart disease), etc. It is the conscientious and explicit use of the current best evidence from systematic research to guide in decision-making and improved patient care by eliminating all gray zones and it is continuously evolving [4–7].

1.1.2 History of Dentistry

Dentistry has evolved over time from a rather barbaric practice to a technologically advanced industry. Now people can undergo dental treatments aided by the state-of-the art technologies in avant-garde infrastructure. Gone are the days of barber and blacksmith dentists and pulling the teeth with dental pelican and other spooky ways of dental treatment. Dentistry has come a long way! (Fig. 1.2)

The art of treating the anomalies pertaining to the teeth and jaws has a long and rich history ranging from toothache being considered as a curse from God to the progression as one of the most advanced and progressive science. Attempts were made to document the journey of this multifaceted profession by Duval, Fitch, Carabelli, Snell, Linderer, Harris, and others; however, a comprehensive documentation was given by Dr. Vincenzo Guerini, of Naples, Italy, who has written a history of dentistry from the earliest times to the beginning of the nineteenth century [8, 9].

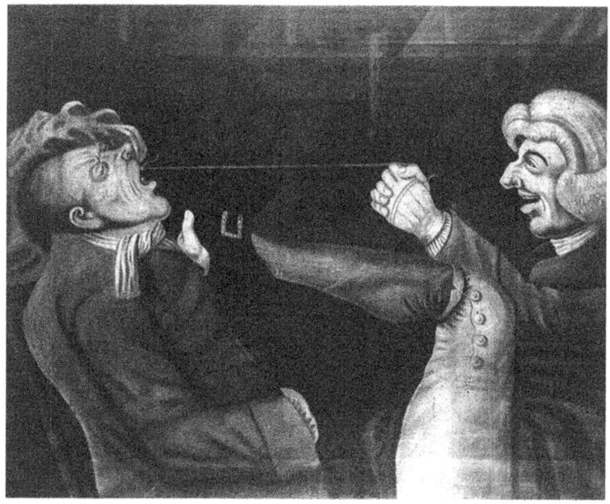

Fig. 1.2 History of dentistry: tooth extraction in the past

1.1.2.1 Dentistry in Antiquity

During these early periods, not many divisions existed in the art of healing. Ailments with reference to teeth and jaws were treated in a general manner, not requiring the services of a specialist. Hippocrates, the Father of Medicine, was the first to give a scientific basis to understanding and treating diseases, before which, anomalies were mainly treated by sacerdotal medicine. Wherein, the cause of diseases was given a superstitious cause requiring sacrifices and rituals to please a supernatural power. One of the earliest cases was found in the Sumerian text which describes "tooth worms" as the cause of tooth decay. The Indus Valley Civilization has yielded evidence of dentistry being practiced as far back as 7000 BC. A site in Mehrgarh indicates that this earliest form of dentistry involved curing tooth-related disorders with bow drill operation, perhaps by skilled bead craftsmen. The earliest dental-filling, made of beeswax, was discovered in Slovenia and dates from 6500 years ago. It is logical that progress in dentistry would go hand in hand with a progress and stability of a particular civilization and the art of dentistry flourished in one of the oldest civilizations, the Egyptians [9].

1.1.2.2 Dentistry in Egyptian History

In Egypt, as in other countries, medicine and dentistry was practiced mainly by the sacerdotal caste, but not all the people in the caste were priests and doctors at the same time. There was a special class of people known as the "Phostophori" whose mission was to cure the sick (Fig. 1.3).

Egyptian skulls dating from 2900 to 2750 BCE contain evidence of small holes in the jaw in the vicinity of tooth's roots. Such holes are believed to have been drilled to drain abscesses. In addition, accounts of dental treatment appear in

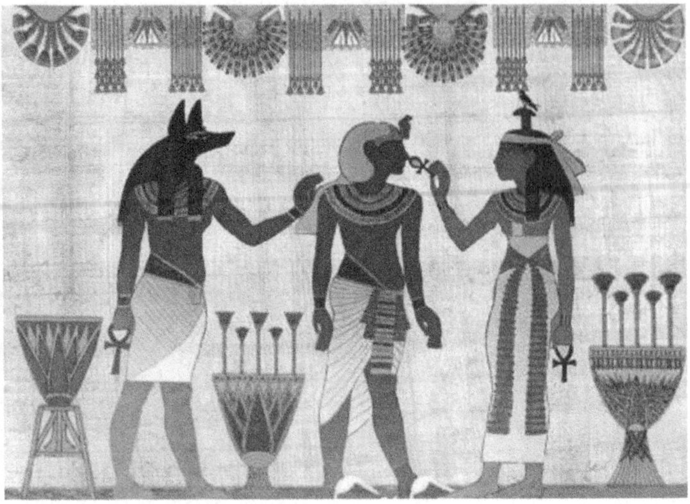

Fig. 1.3 Dentistry in Egyptian history

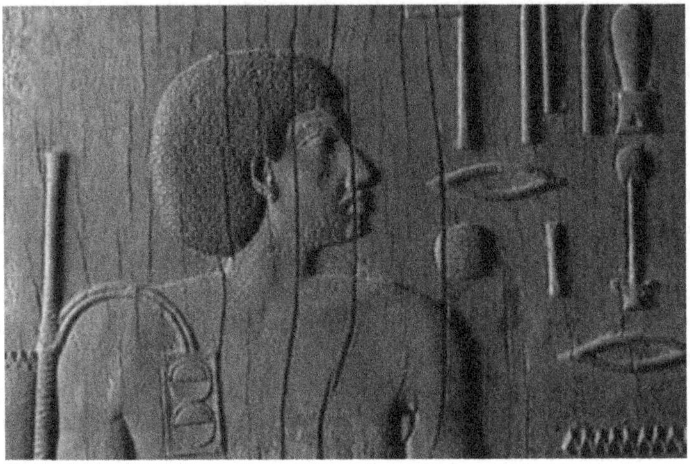

Fig. 1.4 Hesy Re: first dentist

Egyptian scrolls dating from 1500 BCE. It is thought that the Egyptians practiced oral surgery as early as 2500 BCE, although evidence for this is minimal. An early attempt at tooth replacement dates to Phoenicia (modern Lebanon) around 600 BCE, where missing teeth were replaced with animal teeth and were bound into place with cord.

As evidenced by the tomb of "Hesy Re" who is often honored as the first dentist who said "the greatest of those who deal with teeth, and of physicians," this is the first known reference of a person being identified as a dental practitioner [9] (Figs. 1.4 and 1.5).

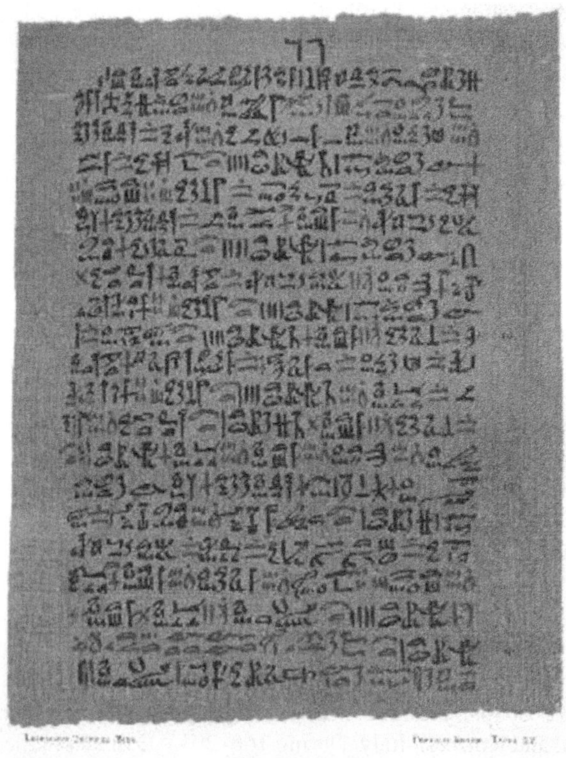

Fig. 1.5 Ebers Papyrus

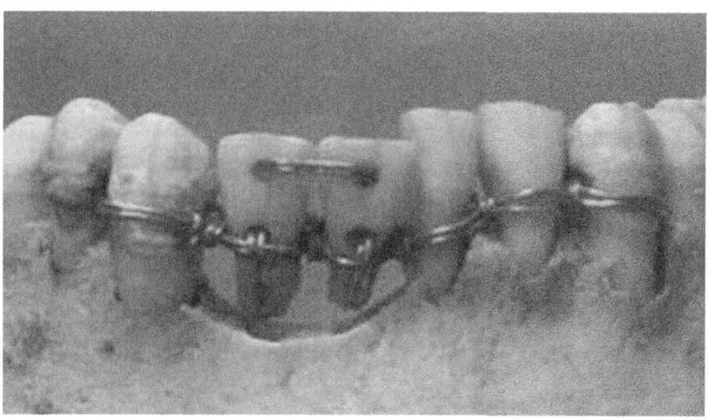

Fig. 1.6 Earliest fixed partial dentures

The Egyptian text known as Ebers Papyrus talks about various ailments of the oral cavity and the remedy for many conditions such as treatment for dental abscess and remedies to strengthen gums for swelling and tooth pain (Fig. 1.6).

There were also attempts at replacing lost teeth, as discovered by archeologists, and teeth united by a gold wire out of which few of those were from other individuals.

1.1.2.3 Dentistry in the Chinese History

There is evidence that the early Chinese practiced some restorative dentistry as early as the year 200 BCE, using silver amalgam as fillings. Oral medicine was part of the regular medical practice in other early Asian civilizations, such as those in India and Japan.

The Chinese called the toothache "ya-tongy" and gave a classification of toothache according to cause. They developed around 18 decoctions for toothache in the form of pills and mouthwashes.

Along with these pills, they also used acupuncture to treat toothache and gum diseases with as much 26 puncture points for toothache and six for gum problems, and some of these points were located at parts of the body distant from the oral cavity. They also used aromatic powdered leaves in a process called "moxibustion" to relieve tooth pain [9] (Fig. 1.7).

1.1.2.4 The Greeks, Romans, and Etruscans

True restorative dentistry began with the Etruscans, who lived around what is today's Central and Northern Italy. During 166–201 AD, they practiced dental prosthetics using gold crowns and fixed bridgework. Numerous dental bridges and partial dentures of gold have been found in Etruscan tombs, which date to about

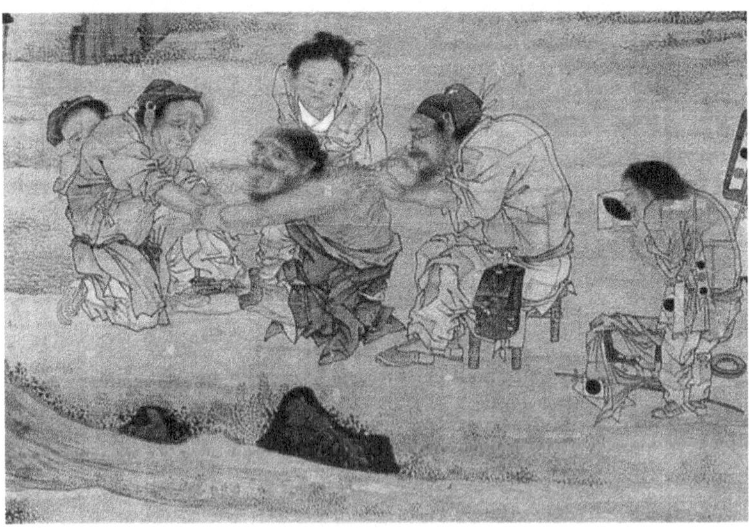

Fig. 1.7 Moxibustion

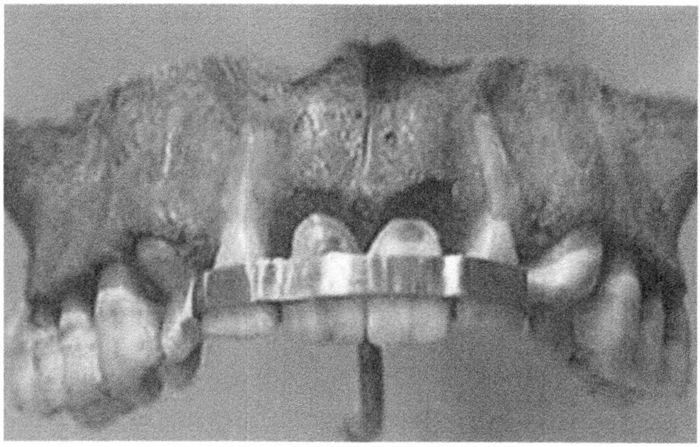

Fig. 1.8 Dental prosthetics using gold

500 BCE. The Romans, who conquered the Etruscans, adopted Etruscan culture, and dentistry became a regular part of Roman medical practice. In 100 BC, Celsus, a Roman medical writer, wrote extensively in his important compendium of medicine on oral hygiene, stabilization of loose tooth, treatments for toothache, teething pain, and jaw fractures (Fig. 1.8).

During the twelfth century BC, a Greek physician named Esculapius was recognized, according to Greek literature, to be the inventor of purgatives and extraction of teeth. Therefore, the first documented origin of dental surgery can be thought of to be from Esculapius. Caelius Aurelianus mentioned of a leaden instrument "plumbeumodontagogoon" used for the extraction of tooth.

During 500–300 BC, Hippocrates and Aristotle wrote about dentistry, including the eruption pattern of teeth, treating decayed teeth and gum disease, extracting teeth with forceps, and using wires to stabilize loose tooth and fractured jaws. The Greeks also practiced some form of oral medicine, including tooth extractions, from the time of Hippocrates, around 400 BCE [9].

1.1.2.5 The Beginnings of a Profession: The Middle Ages

The Arabians certainly had the merit of keeping alive the study of medicine in an age of decadence and barbarism (Fig. 1.9).

Rhazes (or more precisely, Abu Bekr Muhammed ben Zacarjaer Rhazi) stressed upon the need to exhaust every method to cure the teeth before extracting it, hence propagating conservation of tooth structure. To prevent spread of caries, cavities were filled with a cement made of mastic and alum, which is a laudable attempt at stopping progress of tooth decay. Because of the proscription in the Quran, the sacred scripture of Islam, against mutilating the body, surgery was not practiced in Islamic countries. Instead, reliance was placed upon healing using herbs and

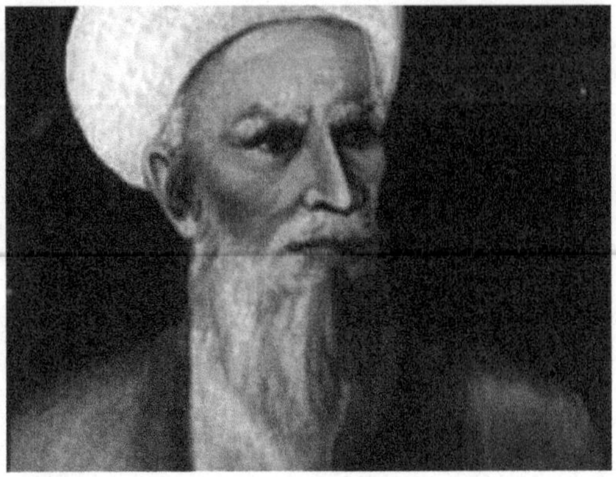

Fig. 1.9 Rhazes

medicines; preventive dentistry through strict adherence to oral hygiene became paramount.

The writings of early Arabic physicians, such as Avicenna and Abū al-Qāsim, show that scaling and cleaning of teeth were practiced. Extractions were rare and were performed only when a tooth had been loosened.

Against periodontitis and the pains produced by it, it was recommended, besides opium, oil of roses, pepper, and honey as well as the scarification of the gums and the application of a leech. If, however, these remedies did not succeed, castoreum, pepper, ginger, storax, opium, and other ingredients were applied to the roots of the teeth. If even this method of cure failed, the root of the diseased tooth was touched with a red-hot iron, or sought to provoke its fall using special medicaments such as coloquintida and arsenic.

Ali Abbas in eight century AD, a Persian physician, wrote about diseases of the tooth and explains the treatment of a periapical lesion by introducing hot needles into the tooth repeatedly until they become cool. He also used chemicals in the tooth like asafetida to devitalize the tooth and relieve the pain. If these methods failed, he would extract the tooth (Figs. 1.10 and 1.11).

Serapion (Jahiak Ebn Serapion), who lived in the tenth century, indicated with great precision the number of dental roots. Against dental pains of phlogistic origin, he recommended bloodletting, purgatives, and many local medicaments. In cases of persistent odontalgia due to caries, he advised the application of opium in the carious cavity. To strengthen loosened teeth, he first employed astringents, and if these are of no use, he bound the loose tooth together to the neighboring healthy ones by means of gold or silver wire.

One of the greatest luminaries of medicine among the Arabs was Avicenna (Ebn Sina). He was born in 980 AD. He was the one who recommended drilling of a tooth with constant pain to remove humors which are accumulated and filling them with medicaments.

Abulcasis (Abul Casem Chalaf Ben Abbas) (1050–1122) was one of the greatest surgeons who recommended cauterization of periapical abscess and fistula as well

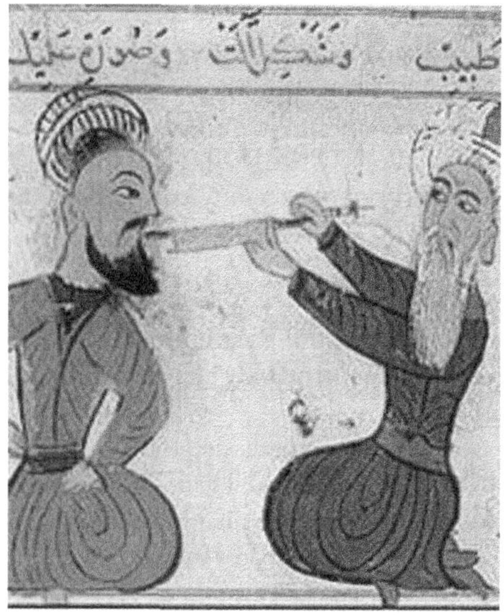

Fig. 1.10 Medieval Islamic dentistry

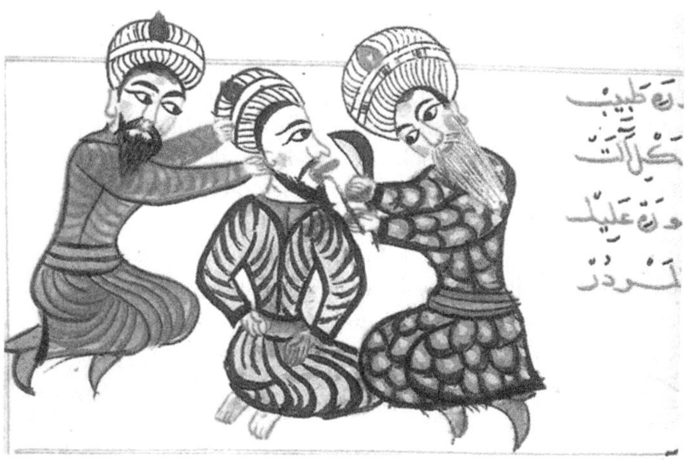

Fig. 1.11 Abulcasis: father of modern surgery

as described the process. His book has one of the first representations of dental instruments. He also advocated ligation of teeth in cases of a blow or fall [9].

- Thirteenth to Fifteenth Centuries

During 1130–1163 AD, a change of guard occurred when a series of Papal edicts prohibited monks from performing any type of surgery, bloodletting, or tooth extraction. After the edicts, barbers assumed the monks' surgical duties. In 1210 AD, a Guild of Barbers is established in France. Barbers eventually evolved into two groups: surgeons, who were educated and trained to perform complex surgical operations, and lay barbers or barber-surgeons, who performed more routine hygienic services including shaving, bleeding, and tooth extraction. However, this was short-lived as in 1400s a series of royal decrees in France prohibited lay barbers from practicing all surgical procedures except bleeding, cupping, leeching, and extracting teeth. In 1530, the *Little Medicinal Book for All Kinds of Diseases and Infirmities of the Teeth* (Artzney Buchlein), the first book devoted entirely to dentistry, was published in Germany [9].

- Sixteenth to Nineteenth Centuries

In the midst of the vigorous intellectual life which characterized the sixteenth century, dentistry too, like many other branches of science, made very notable progress.

Gian Filippo Ingrassia (1510–1580), a distinguished Sicilian anatomist, was one of the first who spoke of the dental germ. He said that the existence of the tooth in proper form depends on a soft dental substance enclosed in the bone, which he considered as a secretion of the latter.

Antonie van Leeuwenhoek (1632–1723), in the year 1683, discovered in the tartar scraped from between the teeth a form of microorganism upon which he laid special stress (Fig. 1.12 and 1.13).

By the 1700s in France, several surgeons were restricting their practice to dentistry, and in 1728 a leading Parisian surgeon, Pierre Fauchard, gathered all that was then known about dentistry in a monumental book, *The Surgeon Dentist*, or *Treatise on the Teeth* (*Le Chirurgien Dentiste*). Fauchard is credited as being the Father of Modern Dentistry because his book was the first to describe a comprehensive system for the practice of dentistry including basic oral anatomy and function, operative and restorative techniques, and denture construction.

Fauchard effectively separated dentistry from the larger field of surgery and thus established dentistry as its own profession. Other surgeons in Germany and France,

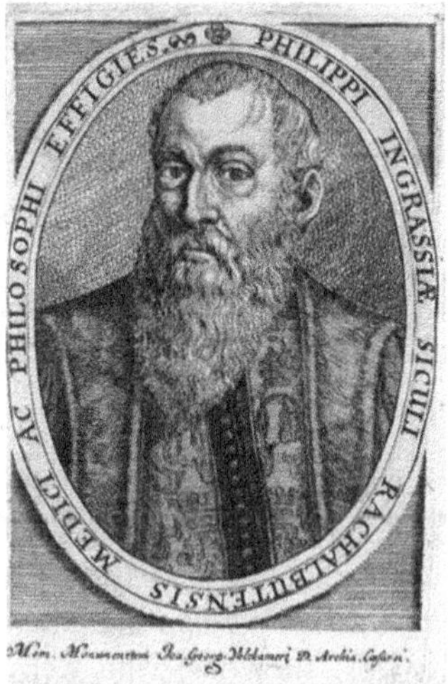

Fig. 1.12 Gian Filippo Ingrassia, the one who first spoke of dental germ

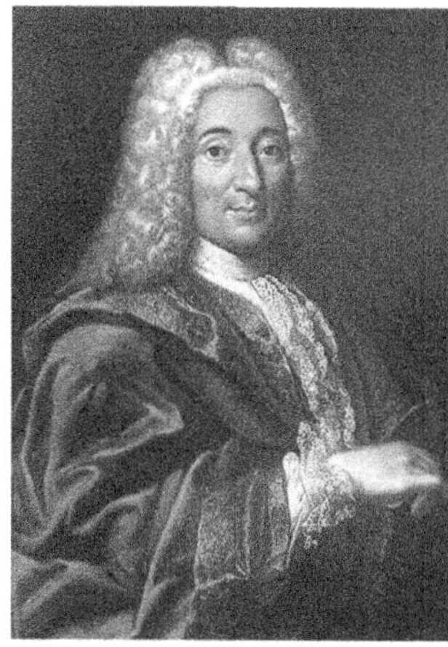

Fig. 1.13 Pierre Fauchard

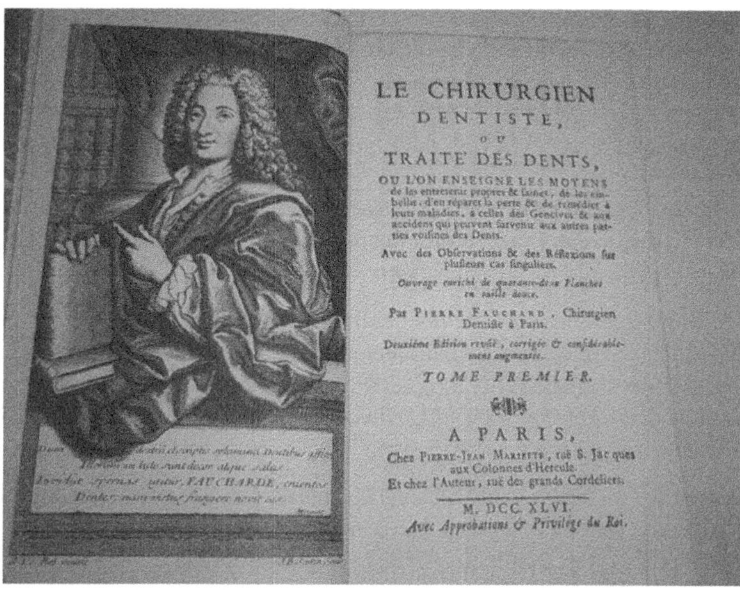

Fig. 1.14 *The Surgeon Dentist*

who made notable contributions to the field of dentistry, readily followed his lead [9] (Fig. 1.14).

In 1746, Claude Mouton described a gold crown and post to be retained in the root canal. He also recommended white enameling for gold crowns for a more aesthetic appearance. In 1789, Frenchman Nicolas Dubois de Chemant received the first patent for porcelain teeth.

In the first known case of postmortem dental forensics, Paul Revere verified the death of his friend, Dr. Joseph Warren, when he identified the bridge that he constructed for him. English dentistry did not advance as far as French dentistry in the eighteenth century. The guild that had united the barbers and surgeons was dissolved in 1745, with the surgeons going their own way. Some barbers continued their dental ministrations and were designated “tooth drawers.” A second group, as a result of the French influence, referred to themselves as “dentists,” while those who did all manner of dentistry were called “operators for the teeth.” The first English book on dentistry, *The Operator for the Teeth*, by Englishman Charles Allen, was published in 1685; however, no other works on English dentistry were published until Thomas Berdmore, dentist to King George III, published his treatise on dental disorders and deformities, in 1768. In 1771 English surgeon John Hunter, famed as the Father of Modern Surgery, published *The Natural History of the Human Teeth*, an outstanding text on dental anatomy. Hunter also pioneered the transplantation of teeth from one individual to another, and, because of his tremendous reputation, this practice was widely adopted. Although tooth transplantation between individuals did not prove successful, it was nevertheless the first attempt to transplant human tissue from one person to another. Later, English dentist Joseph Fox, who served as one of the staff of Guy’s Hospital in London, offered the first observations on what is today recognized as the “rejection phenomenon” of transplants [9].

Following years are marked with greatest discoveries that revolutionized dentistry.

In the year 1790, John Greenwood constructed the first known dental foot engine. In the same year, Josiah Flagg, a prominent American dentist, constructed the first chair made specifically for dental patients.

In 1832, James Snell invented the first reclining dental chair.

In 1833–1850, the Crawcours (two brothers from France) introduce amalgam filling material under the name Royal Mineral Succedaneum.

In 1839, *American Journal of Dental Science*, the world’s first dental journal, began publication.

The need for a professional teaching institution now was of paramount importance, and in the year 1840, Horace Hayden and Chapin Harris founded the world’s first dental school, the Baltimore College of Dental Surgery, and established the Doctor of Dental Surgery (DDS) degree, and in the same year, the first national society of dentists, the American Society of Dental Surgeons, was founded in New York City.

Great new advances in the field came about very quickly at this time. In 1844 American dentist Horace Wells discovered the anesthetic properties of nitrous oxide, which he promptly began using while performing tooth extractions. In 1846 another American dentist, William Thomas Green Morton of Boston, successfully demonstrated in public the effectiveness of ether anesthesia. In 1856 English dentist Sir John Tomes led the formation of the first dental organization in England, the Odontological Society. It was through the activity of this group that the Royal Dental Hospital of London was established in 1858 (Fig. 1.15).

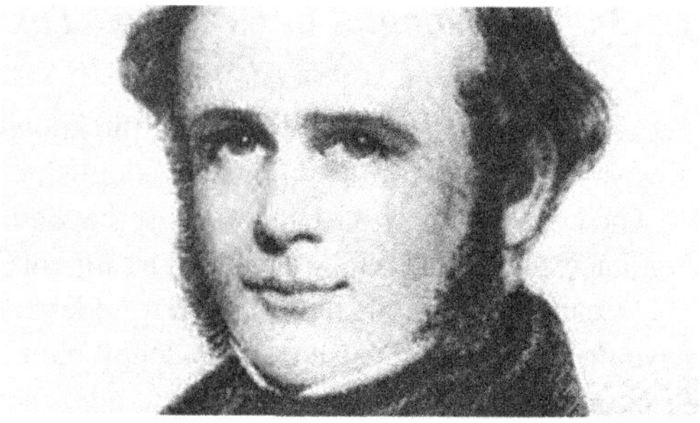

Fig. 1.15 Horace Wells

In 1864 vulcanized rubber was introduced as a substitute for difficult and costly gold dentures, allowing dentists to supply dentures at a lower cost.

In 1871, James B. Morrison patented the first commercially manufactured foot-treadle dental engine. Morrison's inexpensive, mechanized tool supplies dental burs with enough speed to cut enamel and dentin smoothly and quickly, revolutionizing the practice of dentistry. In the same year, American dentist George F. Green received a patent for the first electric dental engine, a self-contained motor and hand piece. In 1890 American dentist Willoughby Dayton Miller published *The Micro-organisms of the Human Mouth*, in which he proposed the theory that dental caries were the result of bacterial activity. Miller's publication led to a tremendous wave of interest in oral hygiene.

In 1895, Wilhelm Roentgen, a German physicist, discovered the x-ray. In 1896 prominent New Orleans dentist C. Edmund Kells took the first dental x-ray of a living person in the United States.

In 1899, Edward Hartley Angle classified the various forms of malocclusion. Credited with making orthodontics into a dental specialty, Angle also established the first school of orthodontics (Angle School of Orthodontia in St. Louis, 1900), the first orthodontic society (American Society of Orthodontia, 1901), and the first dental specialty journal (*American Orthodontist*, 1907).

History has many lessons on what can go wrong, in healthcare, ethics, and the relationship between medicine and society. It also shows how errors can lead into insights. Having knowledge of history gives a better understanding of where we are coming from, thereby giving better clarity of the present and to make educated decisions about the future.

The progress of dentistry into an advanced science is a truly remarkable one. The importance and value of dental art and science as a humane service are well recognized, but we are so accustomed to view the question from the modern standpoint that we overlook the immense work done by our predecessors reaching far back in unbroken line to the mists of time. It was they who laid the cornerstone upon which modern dentistry has been built, and no man can wade through the record of their efforts [9].

1.1.3 Technologies in Dentistry: Through Ages

Technology—the application of scientific knowledge for practical purposes—is and always has been a core component of dentistry.

The consequences of dental disease have plagued humanity throughout history. Our ancestors relied on the tools and treatments available to them and applied available treatment methods based on their understanding. While our ancestors may not have understood the cause of their dental pain, they did find ways to alleviate their discomfort, fight infection, and restore the function of their teeth.

While many of the early beliefs about oral health and some of the treatment methods that transpired may seem barbaric by today's standards, it is interesting to look back through time to see how technologies in dentistry have evolved through the ages [10, 11].

Long before the first comprehensive scientific textbook on dentistry, **Fauchard's *Le Chirurgien Dentiste***, was published in 1728, dentistry was practiced by a variety of craftsmen, primarily barbers, but also wig makers, bloodletters, goldsmiths, and blacksmiths, among others. Yet despite their lack of formal, academic training, these medieval practitioners possessed a distinctive skill-set and used specialized instruments to remove, repair, and replace the hardest tissue in the body [11].

The prominence of the early dental practitioner dates to 1092 when Pope Cyril II of Alexandria decreed that priests and monks would have a new grooming style, a shaven face, and a unique hairstyle. The Pope invited *razor et minutor* (barbers and blood removers) to take up the task. As a result, barbers, and the instruments they used—razor, lance, and scissors—became part of a budding surgical profession and barber-surgeons were created. The use of a scalpel was not far behind [11].

Priests could read medical texts and became physicians but they were not allowed to have blood on their hands and so performed noninvasive interventions. The prohibition against bloodletting and surgery by physician-priests began in 1163 when Pope Alexander III, as part of the Council of Tour, declared: *ecclesia abhorret a sanguine.* Loosely translated it meant *shedding of blood is incompatible with the cleric's holy duty to God.* This was the beginning of the separation of physicians from surgeons, a division that lasted for approximately 800 years. The separation is still visible in the names of venerable institutions that include the words "College of Physicians and Surgeons," for example, in Columbia University College of Physicians and Surgeons and the Royal College of Physicians and Surgeons of Canada [11].

In the early medieval pecking order, barber-surgeons not only were ranked as inferior to formally educated physicians but also, in medieval France, ranked further. The term "Surgeons of the Long Robe" referred to those with some academic training to distinguish them from barber-surgeons, or "Surgeons of the Short Robe." The academically trained surgeons were situated socially between physician-priests at the top and the lowly barber-surgeons. Yet the low status of the barber-surgeons did not prevent kings and queens from using them in military ground battles and on long naval voyages, where they gained experience treating wounded soldiers and sailors. Necessity is the mother of invention and barber-surgeons, who were practical and innovative, responded by making technical advances that went on to have a major impact on society [11].

The first and arguably most prominent of these was **Ambroise Paré** (1510–1590), a barber-surgeon to four French kings, who replaced hot oil cauterization of bleeding wounds with **ligature**. Prior to Paré's innovation, hot boiling oil poured in a wound, without anesthesia, was thought to "purge" gunshot wounds of the presumed poisonous nature of the gunpowder. Many of the soldiers died of shock and sepsis following such excruciating treatment. Paré, known as "the gentle surgeon," invented the use of a **soothing wound dressing**, thereby reducing pain caused by the hot oil and greatly enhancing wound healing and survival. Paré, a Huguenot, was so valuable that his Catholic king, Charles IX, hid him in his bedchamber's closet during the night of August 24, 1572, the date of the "St. Bartholomew massacre," to save him from the murderous rampage. Paré lived to be 80, leading a productive life, adopting new surgical techniques, and developing extraction instruments that we still use today. His ligature of blood vessels and wound dressing technique changed surgery forever [11].

Pierre Fauchard (1678–1761), considered the "**Father of Modern Dentistry**," began as a naval surgeon apprentice to Alexandre Poteleret, surgeon-in-chief to his Majesty's ship in Louis XIV's court. Fauchard witnessed the ravaging effect of scurvy on sailors and in particular on their gums. From this experience and the fact that a lack of funds prevented him from completing formal training in surgery, Fauchard decided to pursue dentistry, which did not require a costly apprenticeship. His experience with Poteleret was more extensive than many practicing dentists had at the time. He became a dental surgeon, one of 21 dentists in Paris at the time. His seminal book, *Le Chirurgien Dentiste*, is a compilation of scientific knowledge of dentistry at the turn of the eighteenth century. The manuscript has many original elements, such as the use of carved ivory obturators with attached teeth for cleft palate, a description of tooth dysplasia, new prosthodontic devices for replacement of missing teeth, and innovation in the type and use of dental instruments [11].

Dr. Horace Wells, a dentist from Connecticut, who was responsible for the use of **anesthesia** in dentistry, had an impact on both medicine and dentistry. He was the first patient to have a tooth extracted under nitrous oxide (NO) anesthesia.

Subsequent technological advances were more incremental and less impactful on other branches of medicine. Nevertheless, these advances helped to make dentistry a highly respected and sought-after profession [11].

- They include the invention of **amalgam** as a material for tooth restoration. Modern amalgams were introduced in the Western world during the early 1800s. French dentist Auguste Taveau developed a dental amalgam in 1816 which contained a small amount of mercury and melted silver coins. In 1826, Taveau used the material as a dental restorative and filler. The mixture had some practical issues because it tended to expand significantly after setting. However, mercury was soft enough to mold to a tooth, and after curing lasted a long time. Two Englishmen, the Crawcour brothers, introduced it in the United States in 1833, amid considerable animosity and professional jealousy from colleagues. Amalgam contained shavings of silver coins, tin, and mercury mixed into a paste. It has been the dental restoration material of choice for the past 180 years, and only recently has it become displaced by advances in highly fracture resistant aesthetic bonding materials.

- In the mid-nineteenth century, **dentures** to replace missing teeth were made of ivory, hippopotamus or human bone, or metal (brass or lead) into which human teeth—along with parts of both horse and donkey teeth—were placed. Starting in 1851, they were replaced by a modern technology, vulcanized rubber, invented by Charles Goodyear, an American, who succeeded in hardening the resin of the rubber tree. An American dentist émigré to Paris, Thomas Evans, first used it as a denture base in 1848.
- **Caries investigation** was significantly advanced when a German-educated, American scientist, Dr. Willoughby D. Miller, described the acid dissolution theory in 1890, who, after extensive research, in 1891 published his epochal work, *The Micro-organisms of the Human Mouth*, which set forth a new theory regarding the cause of dental caries. His postulating a "chemico-parasitic" origin of caries laid the basis for all the modern research in dentistry aimed at wiping this scourge out. Until that time, caries, the most common infectious disease affecting humans, was thought to be caused by worms. Using experimental approaches learned from Dr. Robert Koch, Miller reproduced caries in an environment that simulated the oral cavity while working at the Free University of Berlin. Miller, who is recognized as the first oral microbiologist, was influenced to become a dentist by Dr. Frank P. Abbott, dean of New York College of Dentistry from 1911 to 1924, who was Miller's partner in Berlin and his father-in-law.
- One of the earliest dental tools is a **drill**. The **dental drill** was a major breakthrough in speeding up removal of decayed tissue. The first dental drill appeared in 7000 BC and was an invention of Indus Valley Civilization. The use of modern dental drills started with George F. Green, an American dentist who in 1868 invented the foot pedal operated pneumatic drill and 7 years later patented the electric drill.
- The **pneumatic high-speed air rotor drill** developed by Dr. John Patrick Walsh in 1949 in New Zealand followed the invention of the electric slow-speed drill. Dr. John Borden commercialized the high-speed drill in the 1950s in the United States.
- The **toothbrush** has ancient roots. But the invention of the commercial mass-produced toothbrush is attributed to the Englishman William Addis, who in 1770 came up with the idea while in prison. Using swine bristles thread through holes at the ends of a carved cattle bone, he created the first toothbrush prototype. Once released from prison, he started to mass-produce it. The first three-row bristle toothbrush was invented in 1844, and the first nylon toothbrush was commercialized by DuPont in 1938. The first electric toothbrush was created in 1939.
- **Toothpaste** was invented in 1850. The first toothpaste was based on a formulation of powder or pumice. The invention of modern toothpaste is attributed to the

American dentist Dr. Washington Wentworth Sheffield, who came up with the patent in 1878. He is also credited with placing it into collapsible tubes. The idea came to him while in France observing the tubes used by Parisian painters.

- One of the most significant advances in modern dentistry derives from the use of **dental sealants** to prevent dental decay. In the mid-1960s, Drs. Michael Buonocore and E. I. Cueto introduced the first commercial sealant. The product was based on Dr. Buonocore's work on the development of materials to prevent occlusal caries in posterior teeth. In 1974, Drs. J.W. McLean and A. D. Wilson introduced the glass ionomer cement currently used for fissure sealants.
- The discovery of the role that **fluoride** plays in caries prevention is an achievement that the CDC ranks among the ten greatest public health advances of the twentieth century. Fluoride research had its beginning in 1901, when a young dental school graduate, Frederick McKay, left the East Coast to open a dental practice in Colorado Springs, Colorado. When he arrived, McKay was astounded to find scores of residents with grotesque brownish teeth and began his research, in collaboration with renowned dental researcher Dr. G.V. Black, that led to recognition of fluoride's preventive capabilities, and, 30 years later, to the knowledge that water-borne fluoride can prevent cavities.
- Under the leadership of Dr. H. Trendley Dean at the NIH, the **first major public water fluoridation project** began in Grand Rapids, Michigan, in 1944. The project, which lasted 15 years, showed that the caries rate among Grand Rapids children born after fluoride was added to the water supply dropped more than 60 percent. As a result of their efforts, McKay, Dean, and others helped to transform dentistry into a prevention-oriented profession.
- **Dental implants** made of shells (alloplasts) were used by the Mayan civilization in 600 AD. Dr. Per-Ingvar Brånemark, who is known as the Father of the Modern Dental Implant, made the breakthrough discovery that titanium has a property which allows it to fuse with bone. In the midst of research studies, he realized he could not remove a small titanium cylinder that he had placed in a bone to study how the bone healed through osseointegration.
- **Digital dentistry** refers to a wide scope of technologies and devices—introduced in the past several decades—that incorporate digital or computer-controlled components in contrast to mechanical or electrical devices alone. The digital technologies that might be used in the dental office include CAD/CAM (computer-assisted design, computer- assisted manufacture), cone beam CT, digital x-rays, intraoral camera, dental lasers, and optical scanners, among them.
- One of the most recent technological advances is **Invisalign**, a system that creates a series of computer-generated clear plastic orthodontic realigners to correct slight malocclusions. Invisalign "democratized" orthodontics by making the system available to general practitioners. The 1997 invention is attributed to Zia Chishti and Kelsey Wirth.
- More recently, a new technology developed at the NYU College of Dentistry has been shown to significantly decrease the amount of time required for a patient to wear braces. The process is called *micro-osteoperforation* (popularly known as "**faster braces**"), which involves poking small holes into the patient's gums

tissues of the teeth or their substitutes and the maintenance of the health, function, and aesthetics of these structures and tissues (Adopted May 2018).

Prosthodontics: Prosthodontics is the dental specialty pertaining to the diagnosis, treatment planning, rehabilitation and maintenance of the oral function, comfort, appearance, and health of patients with clinical conditions associated with missing or deficient teeth and/or oral and maxillofacial tissues using biocompatible substitutes (Adopted May 2018).

- **Dental Subspecialties**

General Dentistry: A general dentist is your primary care dental provider. A dentist has many responsibilities including the diagnosis, treatment, care, and management of your overall oral health. Nonmetal fillings, periodontal (gum) care, root canal surgeries, crowns, bridges, and preventive education are some of the services a general dentist provides, among several others.

Cosmetic Dentistry: Cosmetic dentistry procedures include straightening, brightening, reshaping, and even repairing teeth. Cosmetic dentistry focuses on improving a person's smile and may include teeth whitening, dental veneers, dental bonding, white fillings, and invisible braces.

Restorative Dentistry: Restorative dentistry restores your smile and health after tooth damage and disease. Restorative services will improve the structure, health, and appearance of the teeth and mouth for those suffering from ailments.

Geriatric Dentistry: Geriatric dentistry is concerned with the oral health of elderly persons, who usually have significant medical problems and are taking multiple medications. Elderly people often experience symptoms of dental decay and gingival (gum) disorders that differ from symptoms experienced by younger people.

- **Dental Ancillaries**

Dental Hygienist: A dental hygienist is an oral health professional who holds the responsibility of preventing and treating oral diseases. A hygienist cleans teeth, checks the mouth for signs of oral diseases, and performs other preventive dental care.

Dental Assistant: A dental assistant assists with the dentist's efficiency in providing top-quality oral health care. An assistant gives patient care and support as a dentist completes a checkup or procedure [12, 13].

1.2 Oral Health

Oral health means more than "good teeth." It is integral to general health, is essential for well-being, and is a determinant of quality of life (Peterson, 2003) [14]. As put forward by Clark and Vanek in 1984, "Oral health and quality oral health care contribute to holistic health. It should be a right not a privilege" [15].

Oral diseases are among the most common diseases found in humans. Despite their high social and economic burdens, oral diseases receive little attention in many countries and remain a neglected area of international health.

1.2.1 Definition of Oral Health

- **The WHO's Definition of Oral Health**

Oral health is essential to general health and quality of life. It is a state of being free from mouth and facial pain, oral and throat cancer, oral infection, and sores, periodontal (gum) disease, tooth decay, tooth loss, and other diseases and disorders that limit an individual's capacity in biting, chewing, smiling, speaking, and psychosocial well-being (World Health Organization, 2012) [16].

- **According to FDI (World Dental Federation)**

Oral health is multifaceted and includes the ability to speak, smile, smell, taste, touch, chew, swallow, and convey a range of emotions through facial expressions with confidence and without pain, discomfort, and disease of the craniofacial complex (head, face, and oral cavity) (September 6, 2016) [17].

Further attributes of oral health:

- It is a fundamental component of health and physical and mental well-being. It exists along a continuum influenced by the values and attitudes of people and communities.
- It reflects the physiological, social, and psychological attributes that are essential to the quality of life.
- It is influenced by the person's changing experiences, perceptions, expectations, and ability to adapt to circumstances [18].

- **ADA Policy: Definition of Oral Health**

Oral health is a functional, structural, aesthetic, physiologic, and psychosocial state of well-being and is essential to an individual's general health and quality of life [Adopted by the 2014 ADA House of Delegates] [19].

1.2.2 Key Facts of Oral Health (WHO) [16]

- Oral diseases pose a major health burden for many countries and affect people throughout their lifetime, causing pain, discomfort, disfigurement, and even death.
- These diseases share common risk factors with other noncommunicable diseases (NCDs).
- It is estimated that oral diseases affect nearly 3.5 billion people.

- Untreated dental caries (tooth decay) in permanent teeth is the most common health condition according to the Global Burden of Disease 2017.
- More than 530 million children suffer from dental caries of primary teeth (milk teeth).
- Severe periodontal (gum) disease, which may result in tooth loss, is also very common, with almost 10% of the global population affected.
- Oral cancer (cancer of the lip or mouth) is one of the three most common cancers in some countries of Asia and the Pacific.
- Treatment for oral health conditions is expensive and usually not part of universal health coverage (UHC). In most high-income countries, dental treatment averages 5% of total health expenditure and 20% of out-of-pocket health expenditure.
- Most low- and middle-income countries are unable to provide services to prevent and treat oral health conditions.
- Factors contributing to oral diseases are an unhealthy diet high in sugar, use of tobacco, and harmful use of alcohol.
- Most oral health conditions are largely preventable and can be treated in their early stages.

1.2.3 Determinants of Oral Health

The ability to access oral health care is associated with gender, age, education level, income, race and ethnicity, access to medical insurance, and geographic location. Addressing these determinants is key in reducing health disparities and improving the health of everyone. Efforts are needed to overcome barriers to access to oral health care caused by geographic isolation, poverty, insufficient education, and lack of communication skills. Discrepancies in oral health status result from numerous obstacles ranging from social [1], environmental [2], biological, behavioral [3], cultural, economic, and political factors [3, 4] to limited access to oral health-care services, complicated oral health-care systems, a lack of oral health information material [5], and oral heath literacy [6]. The process of acquiring oral health information, appraising its concepts, and applying oral health prevention and treatment plans appropriately requires new skill development called oral health literacy (OHL) [20, 21].

- **Social Determinants**

A confluence of personal, social, economic, and environmental factors contribute to individual and population health. For example, people with a quality education, stable employment, safe homes and neighborhoods, and access to preventive services tend to be healthier throughout their lives. Conversely, poor health outcomes are often made worse by the interaction between individuals and their social and physical environment.

Social determinants are in part responsible for the unequal and avoidable differences in health status within and between communities. Social determinants as a leading health topic recognize the critical role of home, school, workplace, neighborhood, and community in improving health [20, 21].

- **Health Impact of Social Determinants**

Social and physical determinants affect a wide range of health, functioning, and quality of life outcomes. For example:

- Access to parks and safe sidewalks for walking is associated with physical activity in adults.
- Education is associated with:

  Longer life expectancy.
  Improved health and quality of life.
  Health-promoting behaviors like getting regular physical activity, not smoking, and going for routine checkups and recommended screenings.

- Discrimination, stigma, or unfair treatment in the workplace can have a profound impact on health; discrimination can increase blood pressure, heart rate, and stress, as well as undermine self-esteem and self-efficacy.
- Family and community rejection, including bullying, of lesbian, gay, bisexual, and transgender youth, can have serious and long-term health impacts including depression, use of illegal drugs, and suicidal behavior.
- Places where people live and eat affect their diet. More than 23 million people, including 6.5 million children, live in "food deserts"—neighborhoods that lack access to stores where affordable, healthy food is readily available (such as full-service supermarkets and grocery stores) [22] (Fig. 1.16).

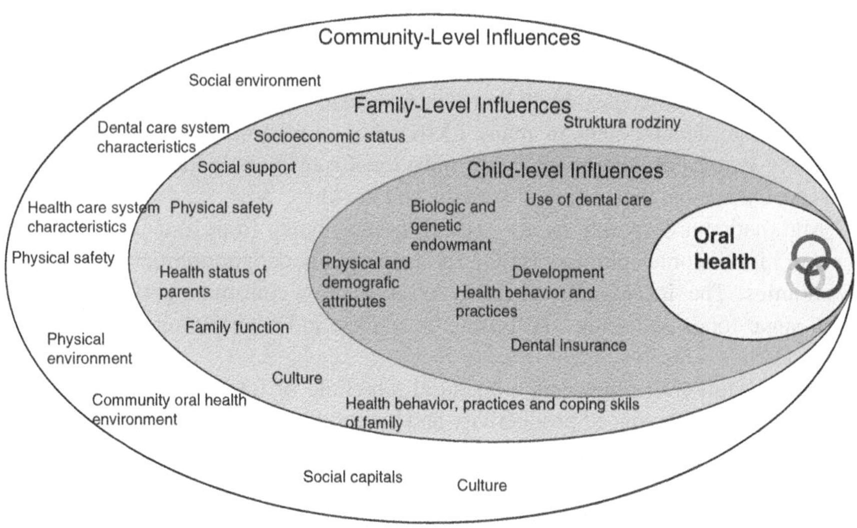

Fig. 1.16 Determinants of oral health

- **Social and Commercial Determinants of Oral Diseases**

The WHO conceptual framework for action on the social determinants of health highlights how structural determinants, such as economic, social, and welfare policies, can generate social hierarchies and influence the socioeconomic status of individuals within societies. Socioeconomic status can then influence health through the circumstances in which people live, work, and age, and their risks for disease. These intermediate determinants include housing and working conditions, social capital, psychosocial factors such as stress and social support, and access to health care [23].

Although the social determinants of health have been well known for some time, the implementation of policies to address these determinants has been slow. The dental public health community has been advocating the importance of integrated upstream and community-based approaches; however, oral health care and approaches to disease prevention still operate to a large extent in a nonintegrated dental silo. Dental policy makers tend to rely on simplistic downstream interventions, in part, because of the dominance of a clinical interventionist philosophy, and because of the challenges of generating evidence of efficacy for the more complex upstream interventions. The biomedical approach to prevention thus prevails and shapes policies that favor the delivery of clinical preventive interventions and chairside oral health advice, rather than population-wide upstream strategies [24].

A number of models have conceptually adapted the WHO social determinants framework for oral health. Additionally, recognition is growing for the need to move from current clinical approaches to policy initiatives that tackle oral health inequalities at the structural level, focusing on the social determinants of health and the risk factors shared between oral diseases and other NCDs, such as free sugar consumption, tobacco use, alcohol consumption, and their wider driving determinants [25].

Globally, a steady overall increase has occurred in the production of sucrose (sourced from sugar beet and sugar cane), the most widely available sweetener since the 1980s. Consequently, in many low- to middle-income countries (LMIC), prevalence of dental caries is increasing at the same time as reported marked increases in the consumption of sugars, including sugary drinks.

Economic development in many LMICs has moved millions out of poverty, resulting in a rapid demographic and nutritional transition characterized by some adverse changes in diet, physical activity, and health.

Multinational corporations are expanding their reach from near-saturated markets in high-income countries (HIC), to also target new opportunities in emerging economies. The increased availability of unhealthy consumer goods, including high-sugar foods and drinks, is shifting behaviors, and contributing to the increase in NCDs.

This overall shift represents a potential minefield of future harms, with poorer health resulting in reduced productivity and burgeoning health-care costs. Buse and colleagues highlighted that "We cannot treat our way out of the NCD epidemic." It calls for a radically different approach.

Hastings has argued that equal concern now needs to be focused on the commercial as well as the social determinants of health [26].

Commercial determinants of health are defined as "strategies and approaches used by the private sector to promote products and choices that are detrimental to health."

In 2013, WHO Director-General, Dr. Margaret Chan, stated that "Efforts to prevent non-communicable diseases go against the business interests of powerful economic operators. In my view, this is one of the biggest challenges facing health promotion" [27].

1.3 Conclusion

Oral diseases are a major global public health problem, having both high prevalence and major negative impacts on individuals, communities, and society. Globally, over 3.5 billion people have oral diseases that are chronic and progressive in nature, starting in early childhood and progressing throughout adolescence and adulthood and into later life. Oral diseases disproportionally affect poorer and marginalized groups in society, being very closely linked to socioeconomic status and broader social and commercial determinants. Increasing consumption of free sugars particularly in LMICs is causing an increase in dental caries, as well as other NCDs such as obesity and diabetes. Dental treatment alone cannot solve this problem. A radically different approach is now needed to tackle this global health challenge [28].

References

1. American Association of Oral and Maxillofacial Surgeons, ADA Definition of Dentistry (1997) http://www.centreoms.com/admin/storage/news/ADA%20Definition%20of%20OMS%20and%20Dentisry.pdf
2. Kamen S, Dorfman J, Connor RA, Ring ME (2018 Jan 4) dentistry. In: Encyclopedia Britannica. https://www.britannica.com/science/dentistry. Accessed 5 December 2021
3. Wikipedia Contributors. Dentistry. In: Wikipedia, The Free Encyclopedia. https://en.wikipedia.org/w/index.php?title=Dentistry; https://en.wikipedia.org/w/index.php?title=Dentistry&oldid=1083404240; https://en.wikipedia.org/w/index.php?title=Dentistry&oldid=1083404240" oldid=1083404240. Accessed 21 Apr 2022
4. Richards D, Lawrence A (1995) Evidence based dentistry. Br Dent J 179:270–273. https://doi.org/10.1038/sj.bdj.4808896
5. Chiappelli F (2019) Evidence-based dentistry: two decades and beyond. J Evid Based Dent Pract 19(1):7–16., issn 1532-3382. https://doi.org/10.1016/j.jebdp.2018.05.001
6. McGlone P, Watt R, Sheiham A (2001) Evidence-based dentistry: an overview of the challenges in changing professional practice. Br Dent J 190:636–639. https://doi.org/10.1038/sj.bdj.4801062
7. Wikipedia Contributors. Evidence-based dentistry. In: Wikipedia, The Free Encyclopedia. https://en.wikipedia.org/w/index.php?title=Evidence-based_dentistry; HYPERLINK https://en.wikipedia.org/w/index.php?title=Evidence-based_dentistry&oldid=1058819440. Accessed 21 Apr 2022

8. American Dental Education Association. History of dentistry. https://www.adea.org/GoDental/Health_Professions_Advisors/History_of_Dentistry.aspx
9. Hussain A, Khan FA (2014) History of dentistry. Arch Med Health Sci [serial online] [cited 2022 Apr 21] 2:106–110. Available from: https://www.amhsjournal.org/text.asp?2014/2/1/106/133850
10. Salgra Dental Group. The evolution of dentistry through ages. https://www.salgradental.com/evolution- dentists-dentistry-through-ages
11. Spielman AI. NYU dentistry. Technology in dentistry, through the ages. https://dental.nyu.edu/aboutus/history-of-nyucd/technology-in-dentistry-through-the-ages.html
12. Webster DDS. 12 types of dental specialities. https://websterdds.com/12-types-of-dental-specialties/
13. National Commission on Recognition of Dental Specialties and Certifying Boards, ADA. https://ncrdscb.ada.org/en/dental-specialties/specialty-definitions
14. WHO. The world oral health report 2003. http://apps.who.int/iris/bitstream/handle/10665/68506/WHO_NMH_NPH_ORH_03.2.pdf;jsessionid=0E7C2787AB704B48CB037350FADE6F25?sequence=1
15. Clinical Guidelines and Integrated Care Pathways for the Oral Health Care of People with Learning Disabilities 2012, http://www.wales.nhs.uk/documents/BSDH_Clinical_Guidelines_PwaLD_2012.pdf
16. World Health Organization. Oral health. https://www.who.int/health- topics/oral--health#tab=tab_1. Accessed 15 Nov 2021
17. FDI, World Dental Federation. https://www.fdiworlddental.org/fdis- definition-oral-health. Accessed 15 Nov 2021
18. Glick M, Williams DM, Kleinman DV, Vujicic M, Watt RG, Weyant RJ A new definition for oral health developed by the FDI World Dental Federation opens the door to a universal definition of oral health. JADA 147(12):915–917. https://doi.org/10.1016/j.adaj.2016.10.001
19. Baiju RM et al (2017) Oral health and quality of life: current concepts. J Clin Diagn Res 11(6):ZE21–ZE26. https://doi.org/10.7860/JCDR/2017/25866.10110
20. Patrick DL et al (2006 June 15) Reducing oral health disparities: a focus on social and cultural determinants. BMC Oral Health 6(Suppl 1):S4. https://doi.org/10.1186/1472-6831-6-S1-S4
21. Healthy People. Determinants of health. https://www.healthypeople.gov/2020/about/foundation-health-measures/Determinants-of-Health
22. Healthy People. Social determinants. https://www.healthypeople.gov/2020/leading-health-indicators/2020-lhi-topics/Social-Determinants
23. Solar O, Irwin A. A conceptual framework for action on the social determinants of health. Social determinants of health discussion paper 2 (policy and practice). http://apps.who.int/iris/bitstream/handle/10665/44489/9789241500852_eng.pdf;jsessionid=9FD7242AB8697358DE3F3D374555FF58?sequence=1
24. Baelum V (2011 Apr 11) Dentistry and population approaches for preventing dental diseases. J Dent 39(Suppl 2):S9–S19. https://doi.org/10.1016/j.jdent.2011.10.015
25. Watt RG (2012 Oct) Social determinants of oral health inequalities: implications for action. Community Dent Oral Epidemiol 40(Suppl 2):44–48. https://doi.org/10.1111/j.1600-0528.2012.00719.x. PMID: 22998304
26. Oral Diseases – a global public challenge. Watt Lancet paper 1 revised. https://discovery.ucl.ac.uk/id/eprint/10079507/3/Watt%20Lancet%20paper%201%20revised%20-%20clean%201%20copy.pdf
27. Mialon M (2020 Aug 17) An overview of the commercial determinants of health. Glob Health 16(1):74. https://doi.org/10.1186/s12992-020-00607-x
28. Peres MA, Macpherson LMD, Weyant RJ, Daly B, Venturelli R, Mathur MR, Listl S, Celeste RK, Guarnizo-Herreño CC, Kearns C, Benzian H, Allison P, Watt RG (2019 July 20) Oral diseases: a global public health challenge. Lancet 394(10194):249–260. https://doi.org/10.1016/S0140-6736(19)31146-8. Erratum in: Lancet. 2019 Sep 21;394(10203):1010. PMID: 31327369

Chapter 2
Introduction to Dental Anatomy and Nomenclature

Dental anatomy is defined here as, but is not limited to, the study of the development, morphology, function, and identity of each of the teeth in the human dentitions, as well as the way in which the teeth relate in shape, form, structure, color, and function to the other teeth in the same dental arch and to the teeth in the opposing arch. Thus, the study of dental anatomy, physiology, and occlusion provides one of the basic components of the skills needed to practice all phases of dentistry [1].

2.1 Formation of the Dentitions (Overview)

Humans have two sets of teeth in their lifetime (heterodont). The first set of teeth to be seen in the mouth is the **primary** or **deciduous** dentition, which begins to form prenatally at about 14 weeks in utero and is completed postnatally at about 3 years of age. In the absence of congenital disorders, dental disease, or trauma, the first teeth in this dentition begin to appear in the oral cavity at the mean age of 6, and the last emerge at a mean age of 28+/−4 months. The deciduous dentition remains intact (barring loss from dental caries or trauma) until the child is about 6 years of age. At about that time, the first **succedaneous** or **permanent** teeth begin to emerge into the mouth. The emergence of these teeth begins the **transition** or **mixed dentition period** in which there is a mixture of deciduous and succedaneous teeth present. The transition period lasts from about 6 to 12 years of age and ends when all the deciduous teeth have been shed. At that time, the permanent dentition period begins. Thus, the transition from the primary dentition to the permanent dentition begins with the emergence of the first permanent molars, shedding of the deciduous incisors, and emergence of the permanent incisors. The mixed dentition period is often a challenging time for the young child because of habits, missing teeth, teeth of distinct colors and hues, crowding of the teeth, and malposed teeth.

K. Shaikh et al., *Artificial Intelligence in Dentistry*,
https://doi.org/10.1007/978-3-031-19715-4_2

The permanent, or succedaneous, teeth replace the exfoliated deciduous teeth in a sequence of eruption that exhibits some variance. After the shedding of the deciduous canines and molars, emergence of the permanent canines and premolars, and emergence of the second permanent molars, the permanent dentition is completed (including the roots) at about 14–15 years of age, except for the third molars, which are completed at 18–25 years of age. In effect, the duration of the permanent dentition period is 12+ years. The completed permanent dentition consists of 32 teeth if none are congenitally missing [1, 2].

2.2 Nomenclature

The first step in understanding dental anatomy is to learn the nomenclature, or the system of names, used to describe or classify the material included in the subject [1].

- **Formulae for Mammalian Teeth**

Human teeth are heterodont and are characterized by four tooth classes: incisors, canines, premolars, and molars. Human teeth are also diphyodont because there are two generations of teeth during a lifespan: 20 deciduous (primary) teeth and 32 permanent teeth. The primary dentition consists of the two types of incisors—central and lateral—canines, and two types of molars, first and second. The primary incisors, canines, and molars get replaced by the successional permanent incisors, canines, and premolars. Permanent dentition also consists of the additional teeth that are three types of molars—first, second, and third.

The denomination and number of all mammalian teeth are expressed by formulae that are used to differentiate the human dentitions from those of other species. The denomination of each tooth is often represented by the initial letter in its name (e.g., I for incisor, C for canine, P for premolar, M for molar). Each letter is followed by a horizontal line and the number of each type of tooth is placed above the line for the maxilla (upper jaw) and below the line for the mandible (lower jaw). The formulae include one side only, with the number of teeth in each jaw being the same for humans [1].

The dental formula for the primary/deciduous teeth in humans is as follows [1, 3, 5] (Fig. 2.1):

This formula should be read as incisors, two maxillary and two mandibular; canines, one maxillary and one mandibular; and molars, two maxillary and two mandibular—or ten altogether on one side, right or left [1, 3, 5].

Fig. 2.1 Dental formula of deciduous dentition

The dental formula for the primary teeth in humans is:

$$I\,\frac{2}{2}\quad C\,\frac{1}{1}\quad M\,\frac{2}{2}\quad = \quad 10$$

The permanent dental formula in humans is:

$$I\frac{2}{2}\;C\frac{1}{1}\;P\frac{2}{2}\;M\frac{3}{3} = 16$$

Fig. 2.2 Dental formula of permanent dentition

Milk teeth

Incisors, I = 2
Canines, C = 1
Molars, M = 2

$$\frac{212}{212} \times 2 = 20$$

Permanent teeth

Incisors, I = 2
Canines, C = 1
Premolar, PM = 2
Molars, M = 3

$$\frac{2123}{2123} \times 2 = 32$$

Fig. 2.3 Formulae for human teeth

A dental formula for the permanent human dentition is as follows [1, 4, 5] (Fig. 2.2):

Premolars have now been added to the formula, two maxillary and two mandibular, and a third molar has been added, one maxillary and one mandibular [1, 5] (Fig. 2.3).

2.3 Tooth Numbering Systems

In 1947 a committee of the American Dental Association (ADA) recommended the symbolic (Zsigmondy/Palmer) system as the numbering method of choice. However, because of difficulties with keyboard notation of the symbolic notation system, the ADA in 1968 officially recommended the "universal" numbering system. A two-digit system proposed by Fédération Dentaire Internationale (FDI) for both primary and permanent dentitions has been adopted by the World Health Organization and accepted by other organizations such as the International Association for Dental Research [1, 5].

- **Universal System**

The American Dental Association recognized the universal numbering system in 1968; however, the name is misleading because it does not have a universal usage. In this system, each tooth in primary dentition is taken one letter, while for permanent dentition, a number is used for each. It is used in the United States due to its simplicity.

- **Symbolic System**

This system was originally proposed by the Hungarian dentist Adolf Zsigmondy, who developed the idea in 1861. Permanent teeth were numbered 1–8, and the primary teeth were numbered using Roman numerals I, II, III, IV, and V from the midline. After that and to make it less confusing, Dr. Corydon Palmer who is an American dentist changed the Roman numerals of the primary teeth to A, B, C, D, and E. Thus, it is usually referred to as the Zsigmondy/Palmer notation system. In this system, the arches are divided into four quadrants.

The Palmer notation consists of a symbol (┘ └ ┐ ┌) designating in which quadrant the tooth is found and a number indicating the position from the midline. Permanent teeth are numbered 1–8, while deciduous teeth are indicated by letters A to E. This numbering system presents difficulties when an appropriate font is not available for keyboard recording of these notations.

- **FDI System**

The Fédération Dentaire Internationale (FDI) recognized and approved a two-digit system for both primary and permanent dentitions. This system has been adopted by the World Health Organization (WHO) and is accepted by other organizations and in research and public health journals. For the primary teeth, the first digit is from 5, 6, 7 and 8 which denotes the quadrant of the oral cavity starting from the upper right quadrant and moving in a clockwise direction. While for permanent dentition, the first digit is from 1, 2, 3, and 4. The second digit in the FDI system refers to the number of the tooth whether primary or permanent incisors. Hence, the right and left maxillary central incisors of the primary dentition would be numbered 51 and 61, respectively, and the permanent right maxillary central incisor is indicated by the two-digit 11 (pronounced one-one, not eleven). FDI is considered the international system and all practitioners should know how to use the FDI system (Figs. 2.4, 2.5, 2.6, and 2.7).

2.4 Development and Eruption of Teeth

Knowledge of the development of the teeth and their emergence into the oral cavity is applicable to clinical practice, anthropology, demography, forensics, and paleontology [1].

Historically, the term *eruption* was used to denote the tooth's emergence through the gingiva, but then it became more completely defined to mean continuous tooth movement from the dental bud to occlusal contact. Emergence of the primary dentition takes place between the sixth and thirtieth months of postnatal life. Permanent

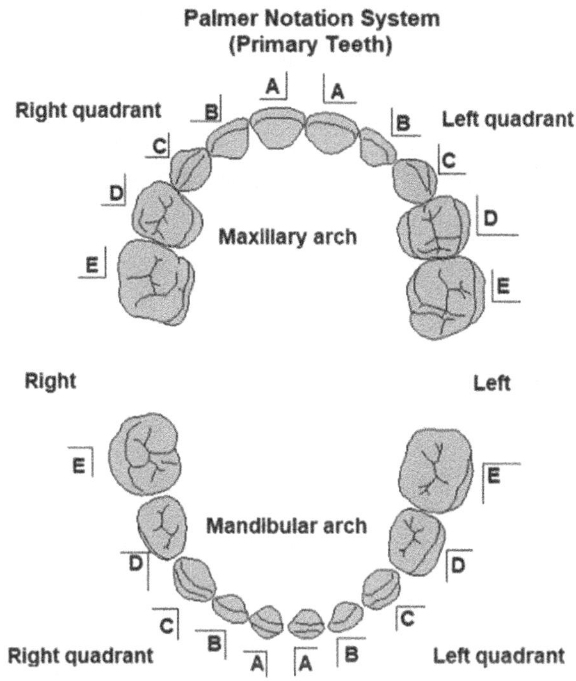

Fig. 2.4 Palmer notation system (primary teeth)

teeth typically begin erupting around age 6, although they may appear earlier or later, usually in correlation with when the primary teeth came in. Most of the permanent teeth begin to erupt several weeks after the corresponding baby teeth fall out; however, while there are 20 baby teeth, ultimately 32 permanent teeth will emerge (16 in each jaw). Twelve of these teeth do not replace baby teeth.

Permanent teeth grow beneath the gingiva in the jawbone under the existing primary teeth. Over time, the root of each primary tooth begins to resorb (dissolve), and the crown, or top, of the incoming permanent tooth forms in the space where the root of the primary tooth breaks down. Then it becomes loose as the permanent tooth continues to form, eventually pushing its way through the pathway left by the lost primary tooth. Because the jawbone grows faster than the rest of the face, it will eventually be able to accommodate 32 permanent teeth where the 20 primary teeth began [1, 2, 5] (Figs. 2.8 and 2.9).

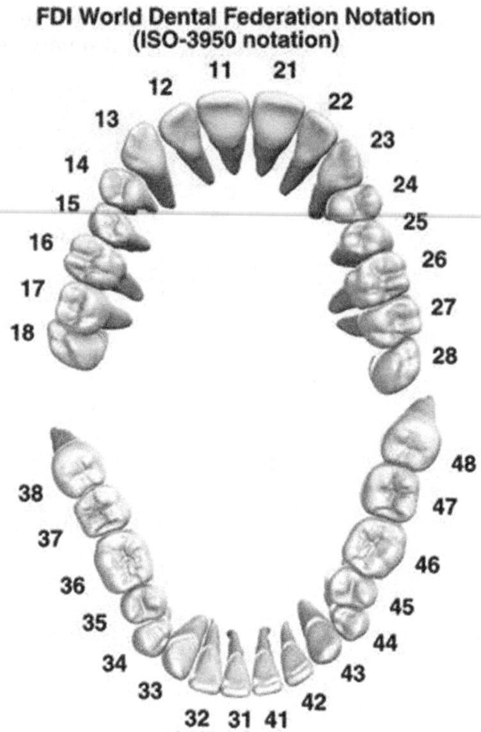

Fig. 2.5 FDI notation system (primary teeth)

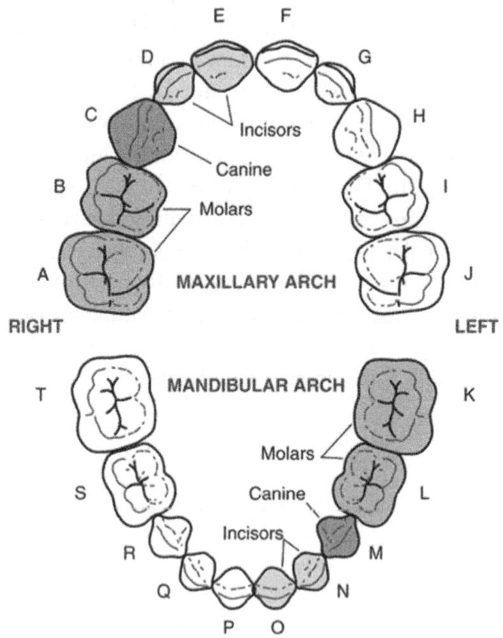

Fig. 2.6 Universal numbering system (primary teeth)

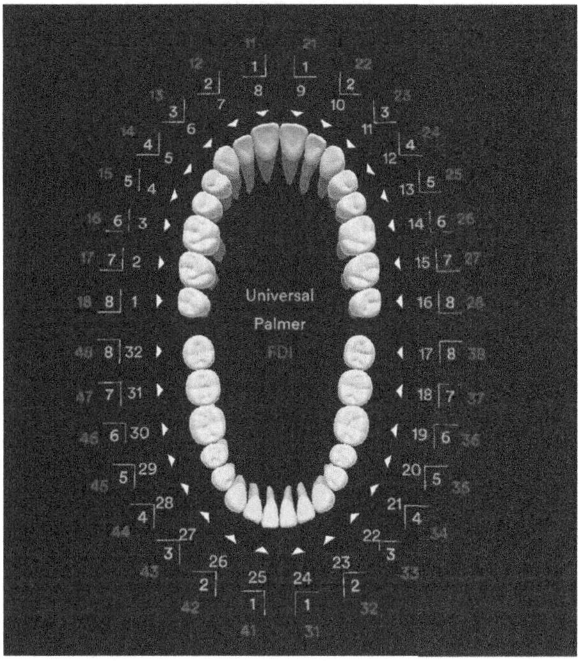

Fig. 2.7 Tooth notation system (permanent teeth)

2.4.1 Chronology Table of Primary and Permanent Dentition (Tables 2.1 and 2.2)

2.5 Anatomy of Teeth (Overview)

The anatomy of a tooth divides into two main sections: the crown and the root. The crown of the tooth is what is visible in the oral cavity, and the root of the tooth is embedded into the bony ridge of the upper and lower jaws called the alveolar process via attachment to the periodontal ligament. The gingiva covers the border of the alveolar process that is adjacent to the teeth. The cementoenamel junction is the anatomical boundary between the enamel-covered crown and cementum-covered root. Dentin makes up the core of the entire tooth that surrounds the pulp, which contains the neurovascular structures. The apical foramen at the root apex is where the neurovascular structures enter the tooth and travel up the root canal to the expanded pulp chamber of the crown. The roots of the tooth vary depending on the type of tooth. The molars typically have three roots: a lingual root on the lingual aspect and a mesiobuccal root and distobuccal root on the buccal aspect. The crown of the tooth has five surfaces. The surface facing the lip or cheek is called the facial surface for incisors and canines and buccal surfaces for premolars and molars. The surface facing the inside of the mouth is referred to as the palatal surface in the

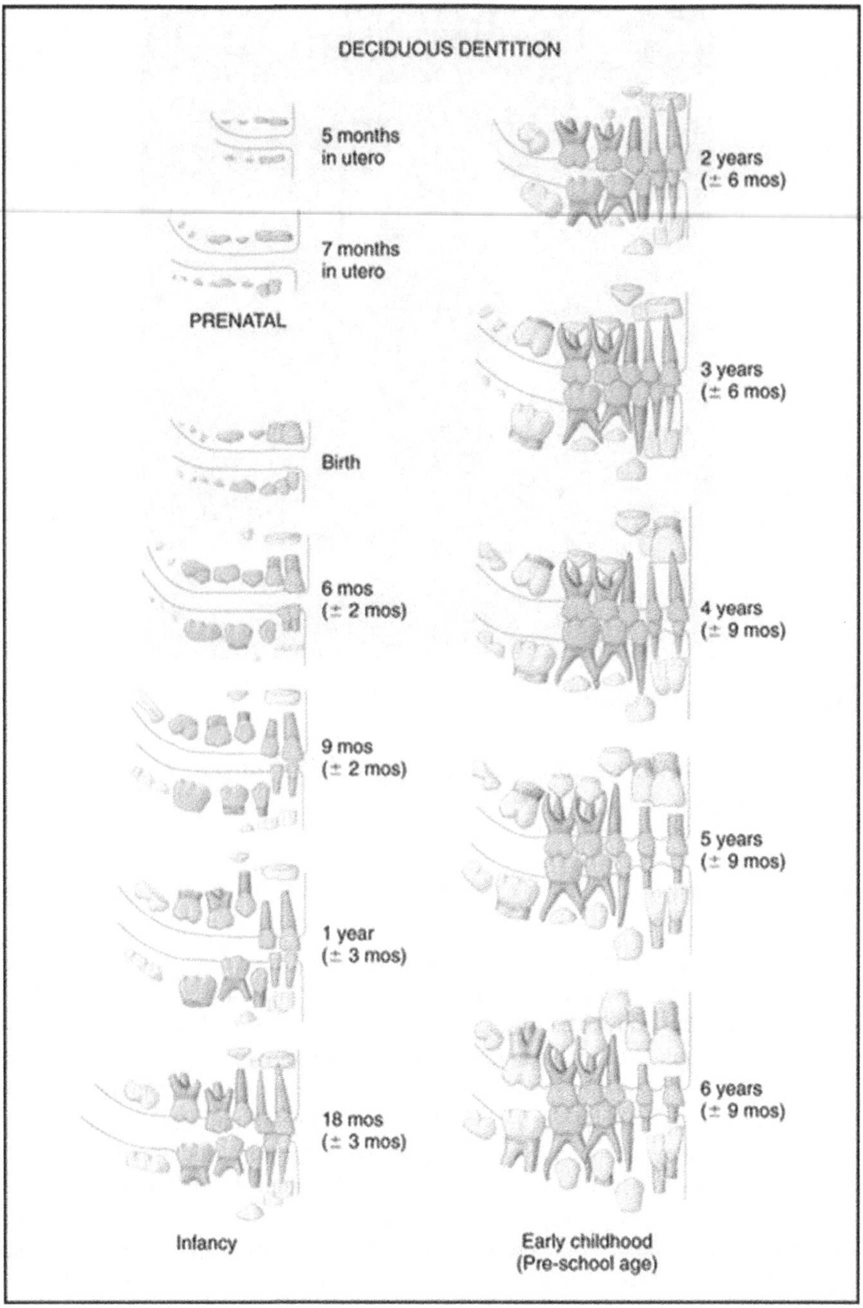

Fig. 2.8 Development of the human dentition to the sixth year. The primary teeth are the darker ones in the illustration (From Schour L, Massler M: The development of the human dentition, *J Am Dent Assoc* 28:1153, 1941). (Image source [1])

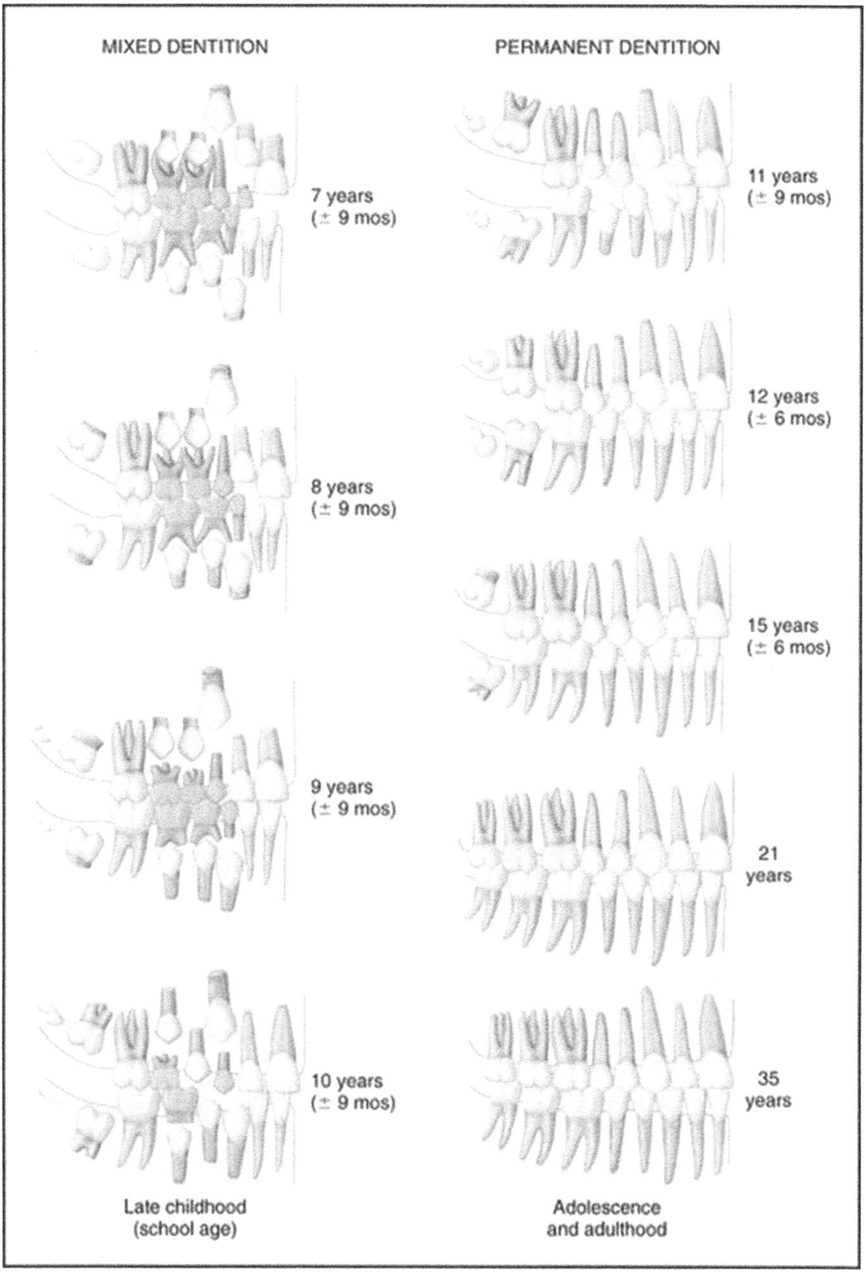

Fig. 2.9 Development of the human dentition from the seventh year to maturity. Note the displacement of the primary teeth (From Schour L, Massler M: The development of the human dentition, *J Am Dent Assoc* 28:1153, 1941). (Image source [1])

Table 2.1 Chronology of primary teeth

Tooth		First Evidence of Calcification (Weeks in Utero)	Crown Completed (Months)	Eruption (Mean Age) (Months)	Root Completed (Years)
Upper					
i1	E, F	14	1½	10	1½
i2	D, G	16	2½	11	2
c	C, H	17	9	19	3¼
m1	B, I	15	6	16	2½
m2	A, J	19	11	29	3
Lower					
i1	P, O	14	2½	8	1½
i2	Q, N	16	3	13	1½
c	R, M	17	9	20	3¼
m1	S, L	15½	5½	16	2¼
m2	T, K	18	10	27	3

Maxillary Teeth
Right A B C D E | F G H I J Left
T S R Q P | O N M L K
Mandibular Teeth

i1, Central incisor; i2, lateral incisor; c, canine; m1, first molar; m2, second molar.
*Universal numbering system for primary/deciduous dentition; see Chapter 1. See Tables 2-3 and 2-4 for detailed presentation of the data.

Image source [1]

maxilla and the lingual surface in the mandible. The surfaces referring to the boundaries of adjacent teeth are called mesial and distal. Mesial refers to the surface closer to the midline of the face, and distal refers to the surface away from the midline of the face. The biting surface is called the occlusal surface [1, 6].

The structure of a tooth is made up of specialized tissues that allow it to survive the forces of mastication while maintaining retention in the oral cavity. Enamel is the hardest tissue in the body and serves as a protective outer covering for the tooth crown. Enamel consists of 96% mineral by weight primarily of a complex, highly organized structure of carbonate-substituted hydroxyapatite mineral arranged in

Table 2.2 Chronology of permanent teeth

Tooth		First Evidence of Calcification	Crown Completed (Years)	Emergence (Eruption) (Years)
I1	8, 9	3-4 mo	4-5	7-8
I2	7, 10	10-12 mo	4-5	8-9
C	6, 11	4-5 mo	6-7	11-12
P1	5, 12	1½-1¾ yr	5-6	10-11
P2	4, 13	2-2¼ yr	6-7	10-12
M1	3, 14	At birth	2½-3	6-7
M2	2, 15	2½-3 yr	7-8	12-13
M3	1, 16	7-9 yr	12-16	17-21
		Maxillary Teeth		
		Right 1 2 3 4 5 6 7 8 | 9 10 11 12 13 14 15 16 Left		
		32 31 30 29 28 27 26 25 | 24 23 22 21 20 19 18 17		
		Mandibular Teeth		
I1	24, 25	3-4 mo	4-5	6-7
I2	23, 26	3-4 mo	4-5	7-8
C	22, 27	4-5 mo	6-7	9-10
P1	21, 28	1¾-2 yr	5-6	10-12
P2	20, 29	2¼-2½ yr	6-7	11-12
M1	19, 30	At birth	2½-3	6-7
M2	18, 31	2½-3 yr	7-8	11-13
M3	17, 32	8-10 yr	12-16	17-21

I1, Central incisor; *I2*, lateral incisor; *C*, canine; *P1*, first premolar; *P2*, second premolar; *M1*, first molar; *M2*, second molar; *M3*, third molar.
*See Tables 2-3 and 2-4 in Tooth Formation Standards for detailed presentation of the data.

Image source [1]

interlocking prisms giving it its characteristic strength. Dentin is the most plentiful tissue in a tooth, and it is mostly responsible for the size and shape of a tooth.

Dentin consists of 60% mineral by weight and 20% organic component arranged in a complex organization of tubules filled with fluid. Dentin's structure can flex and absorb force allowing it to function as a substructure for enamel. The pulp is a specialized tissue at the core of the tooth that contains blood vessels, nerves, odontoblasts, fibroblasts, and an extracellular matrix providing the tooth with neurosensory function and reparative potential. Cementum is the specialized hard tissue covering the tooth root that connects to the periodontal ligament attached to the alveolar bone; this works as an attachment system to hold the tooth in place under physiological loads of mastication [1, 6] (Fig. 2.10).

The periodontal ligament connects the tooth to the alveolus, provides support to withstand the forces of mastication, and contains sensory fibers for proprioception. The tooth root is embedded within the alveolus, which is composed of both cortical and cancellous bone. Along the lip or cheek (labial or buccal) aspect of the alveolus, the bony plate is generally thinner compared to the aspect that faces the tongue (lingual or palatal).

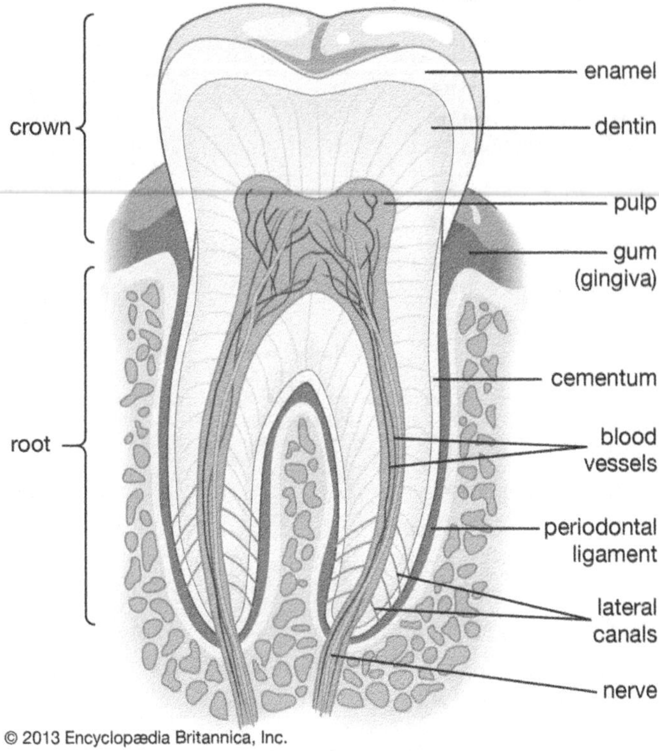

Fig. 2.10 Anatomy of tooth. (Image source: Britannica)

The oral mucosa covering the upper part of the alveolar ridge and immediately surrounding an erupted tooth is referred to as the gingiva, and it forms a tight protective cuff around the cementoenamel junction (neck) of the tooth. The potential space between the gingival cuff and the enamel of the crown is called the gingival crevice. The conglomeration of tissues that surround and serve to support the tooth is collectively known as the periodontium [1, 7] (Fig. 2.11).

2.6 Applications of Technology in Dental Nomenclature and Anatomy

Development and evolution of human teeth is a complicated process and till now it is not completely well understood. The advancement and development of new technologies, such as genomic analysis implementing modern technologies such as next-generation sequencing (NGS) and other "omics technologies," has boosted molecular understanding of tooth development. Information retrieved from these

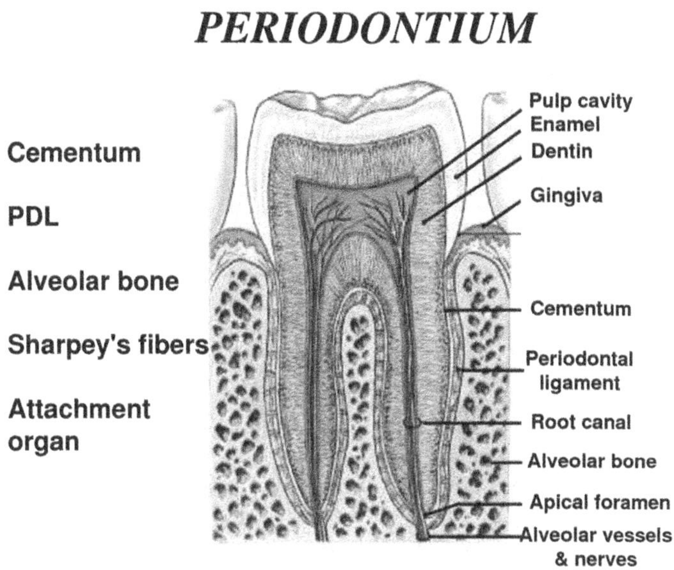

Fig. 2.11 The periodontium components. (Image source [8])

technologies represents a substantial increase in data that need to be selected, analyzed, and integrated. There is no doubt that without the advances of AI technology, our understanding of tooth development will be so limited. The power of AI technology is the ability of AI-based technology to extract, analyze, and process large and complex data. For molecular biology research, AI can help in DNA sequencing, RNA sequencing, prediction of the binding sites of transcription factors, prediction of the protein structure, prediction of DNA-RNA interaction, and protein-protein interaction and other unlimited functions in the field of biomedical science.

Using AI-based technology has increased our understanding about how amazing this structure is. The development of the mammalian teeth is a very complex process that results from sequential and reciprocal interaction between oral ectodermal and the underlying mesenchymal tissues of the first branchial arch [9]. This interaction is completely under the genetic control of many signaling molecules, for example, sonic hedgehog (Shh), fibroblast growth factor (FGF), bone morphogenetic protein (BMP) [10], and Wingless type (Wnt) [11]. These signaling molecules are secreted first by the oral epithelium. They then diffuse into the underlying ectomesenchyme and induce expression of the transcription factors Msx-1, Msx-2, Lef-1, and Dlxs [12]. This reciprocal interaction between these two opposing sets of molecules (signaling molecules and transcription factors) regulates and controls the morphodifferentiation and cytodifferentiation of different cells of the tooth germ [13, 14].

As a result of this continuous interaction, a tooth germ is formed that includes the enamel organ, dental papilla, and dental follicle. The tooth germ goes through different morphological stages until the tooth is completely formed. First, the oral ectoderm thickens to form the primary epithelial band that gives rise to the dental lamina. The dental lamina subsequently invaginates into the ectomesenchyme corresponding to the positions of the future teeth. It then proceeds to form a bud, cap, and finally bell-shaped structures [9, 11].

Although these three structures (enamel organ on the one hand and dental papilla and follicle on the other) have different embryological origins and different fates, they all act in an orchestrated fashion devoted to the formation of different shapes of teeth (morphogenesis) and their correct position in the jaws (patterning).

Furthermore, advances of AI-based technology enhanced our knowledge about genetic mutations that cause developmental anomalies such as hypodontia or anodontia. For example, mutations in genes that are expressed at the early stages of tooth development, such as Msx-1, Pax-9, and Lef-1, cause development blockage either before dental lamina formation and the bud stage or before morphogenesis of the bud into cap stage, thus highlighting their importance in the tooth development process [14]. Also, abnormalities in all these signaling pathways result in morphological variability and dental malformations which may be of significant clinical importance.

Using AI in automatic detection and numbering human teeth on different types of radiographs have been proposed by many studies. The main reason for that is trying to decrease human errors and also proposing automated solutions that might support dentists in their clinical decision-making and saving time in daily practice. For example, a recent study was conducted by Bilgir et al., in 2021 in 2021, trying to use convolutional neural network (CNN) model with 22 deep layers for detection and numbering of teeth in comparison to human expert [15]. The study showed that deep CNN can be used for automatic tooth detection and numbering with high accurate rate (95.5%) and precision rate (96.5%) in comparison to human experts. The study also suggested that different types of AI-based technology and systems can be used to support clinicians in detecting and numbering teeth on panoramic radiographs and may eventually replace evaluation by human observers and improve performance in the future [15]. Another study conducted by Lin et al., in 2010, aimed to develop a system based on a pattern recognition which is AI-based technology for dental classification and numbering system [16]. The study used intraoral bitewing radiographs for training AI machines to be used for the purpose of segmentation, classification, and numbering of teeth. The study reported that AI-based machines can show an accuracy rate of 95.7% for automated numbering and classification teeth [16].

Other two studies used deep learning technology for automated detection and numbering of teeth. The first study was conducted by Chen et al., in 2019 [17], who used dental periapical films to train machines and reported precision rate more than 90% when it is compared to human experience as ground truth. The second study was conducted by Tuzoff et al., in 2019, which was focusing on using deep learning for tooth detection and numbering using 1352 panoramic radiographs to provide automated dental charting according to the FDI two-digit notation. Teeth numbering method was based on the VGG-16 convolutional architecture. The main idea was to test the possibility to achieve numbering of maxillary and mandibular teeth in a single image using the power of the AI deep learning technology [18]. The study demonstrated the capability of CNN machine to have a close sensitivity and precision rates for automatic tooth numbering comparable to grounded truth by 0.9941 and 0.9945, respectively [18].

2.7 Developmental Disturbances of Teeth

Odontologist must be able to identify and recognize normal anatomy of the teeth and also any variations and abnormalities. Identification of the normal size, shape, and number of teeth is considered basic skills for any dentist. In addition, variations in the morphology as well as the structure of the teeth, whether it is common or rare, should be recognized by any dental professionals. Multiple factors are responsible for successful tooth development including genetic and environmental factors. Any interruption during odontogenesis can lead to developmental disturbances in the size, shape, number, and structure of teeth [19].

2.7.1 Developmental Disturbances in Size of Teeth

Several etiological factors have been identified causing teeth size variation in both permanent and primary dentitions including genetic, gender, race, and environmental.

There are several conditions and variations of tooth size including the following:

- **Microdontia**

  Microdontia is an anomaly in which teeth appear smaller than the normal [19]. Microdontia affects few teeth and is rarely seen in a generalized pattern. It is predominantly seen in females than males with a prevalence rate of 1.5–2% [17]. Microdontia can be classified into true, relative, and isolated/localized microdontia.

- *True generalized microdontia* is rare in which all the teeth are smaller than normal. It is usually associated with syndromes such as pituitary dwarfism, Down syndrome, oro-facial-digital syndrome, or oculo-mandibulo-facial syndrome although a few non-syndromic cases have also been reported [17, 20].
- *Relative generalized microdontia* is when the mandible and maxilla have a relatively larger size giving an impression of teeth appearing smaller [17].
- *Isolated microdontia or localized microdontia* affecting single tooth, also called as localized microdontia, is a common condition predominantly affecting the maxillary lateral incisor and third molar. The maxillary lateral incisors manifest a conical or peg shape where the mesial and distal surfaces converge incisally forming a cone-shaped tooth [21].

- **Macrodontia**

Macrodontia refers to a tooth or a group of teeth that are larger than normal. Like microdontia, macrodontia can also be classified as true generalized macrodontia, relative generalized macrodontia, and isolated or localized macrodontia [22]. Mutation in any of the genes of the HOX family, transcription factor Pax 9, or disruption in the signaling pathways that play an important role in odontogenesis may result in macrodontia [22]. Macrodontia is predominantly seen in children between ages 8 and 13 with a prevalence rate of 0.03–1.9% and has male predilection [22]. Teeth that are altered by fusion and gemination should not be confused with macrodontia.

- *True generalized macrodontia* is rare in which all the teeth are larger than normal. It is usually associated with conditions such as pituitary gigantism, KBG syndrome, hemifacial hyperplasia, and Klinefelter's syndrome [22].
- *Relative generalized macrodontia* is when the mandible and maxilla have a relatively smaller size giving an illusion of teeth appearing larger than normal [23].
- *Isolated macrodontia or macrodontia* affecting single tooth also called as localized macrodontia is highly unusual. Bilateral macrodontia is observed in incisors, mandibular premolars, and third molars [24].

Microdontia and macrodontia can pose aesthetic concerns and functional difficulties. Treatment modalities for microdont and macrodont teeth could vary from orthodontic treatment to restorative treatments (composite or porcelain veneers) and extractions depending upon each case scenario [25].

2.7.2 *Developmental Disturbances in Number of Teeth*

- **Anodontia**

Anodontia is described as complete agenesis of the dentition. True anodontia usually involves permanent dentition more than the deciduous dentition; however, association between missing primary and permanent dentitions has been reported [26]. True anodontia or congenitally missing teeth is classified into two types: total and partial. Total anodontia is highly unusual and is most likely seen in association with hereditary ectodermal dysplasia [19, 26]. Partial anodontia also referred to as hypodontia or oligodontia is the congenital absence of one tooth or more teeth. Third molars, maxillary lateral incisors, and maxillary or mandibular second premolars are the most common missing teeth unilaterally or bilaterally. Several factors such as thalidomide treatment, chemotherapy, and radiotherapy in early infancy and trauma to the alveolar process have been implicated in the development of hypodontia. The most frequently reported genes associated with hypodontia are Msx1 (muscle segment homeobox 1), AXIN2 (axis inhibition protein 2), PAX9 (paired box gene 9), and EDA (ectodysplasin A). Treatment attributes for patients with hypodontia are challenging although implant treatments have shown promising results [27].

- **Supernumerary Teeth**

Supernumerary teeth, also known as hyperdontia, refer to the presence of an additional tooth or teeth to the existing series of teeth. Supernumerary teeth can be unilateral or bilateral, and it can be present in one or both jaws with the anterior maxilla as a predominant region [28]. The most accepted theory for the occurrence of supernumerary teeth is hyperactivity of the dental lamina [29]. Supernumerary teeth have a prevalence rate of 0.2–3% in the primary and permanent dentition with male predominance [29]. Supernumerary tooth can be present in different locations with different names, for example, an extra tooth that is located between the two maxillary central incisors is called a "mesiodens" and when present adjacent or distal to the molar region is called a distomolar or paramolars (lingually or buccally). Single supernumerary tooth is classified as conical, odontoma (complex and compound), tuberculate, and supplemental (non-syndromic). Multiple supernumerary teeth are associated with cleft lip and palate, cleidocranial dysplasia, and Gardner syndrome [30]. It must not be any confusion between supernumerary teeth with dental transpositioning, a pattern of abnormal eruption. Supplemental teeth are excessive teeth that resemble the morphology of normal teeth. The most commonly occurring supplemental teeth are the permanent maxillary lateral incisor [28].

- **Natal and Neonatal Teeth**

Natal teeth are present at birth which develop and erupt during the intrauterine life, while neonatal teeth erupt during the first month of life, creating a disturbance in physiological chronology [31]. Studies have reported a higher incidence rate of natal teeth than neonatal teeth with a ratio of 3:1 [31]. Teeth that erupt after 30 days of life but within 3.5 months are called as "early infancy teeth." Eighty-five percent of natal teeth are mandibular incisors [32]. The etiology of natal and prenatal teeth is still unknown although several factors such as infections, malnutrition, hormonal stimulation, hereditary transmission, and superficial positioning of the tooth germ have been implicated as plausible factors [33].

Natal and neonatal teeth are composed of enamel and dentin with or without the presence of pulp or root formation [33]. They appear as small conical-shaped teeth of yellow-brown or a whitish opaque color with grade III mobility [31]. Ulceration of the ventral surface of the tongue also called as Riga-Fede disease, tooth aspiration, and difficulty in breastfeeding are few of the complications associated with the presence of natal and neonatal teeth [34]. Due to the potential complications, extraction within the 7th–25th day of birth is usually the choice of treatment with prophylactic administration of vitamin K [35].

2.7.3 Developmental Disturbances in Shape of Teeth

- **Gemination**

Gemination, also called as double tooth, has been described as an attempt of a single tooth germ to divide resulting in the formation of a complete or partial bifid crown usually with a common root and root canal [36]. It is a common dental anomaly seen in both deciduous and permanent dentitions with a predilection toward anterior and maxillary region [36]. In gemination the tooth count is normal when compared to fusion.

- **Fusion**

Fusion is defined as the union of two normally separated tooth germs resulting in the formation of a joined tooth [36]. It is a common dental anomaly seen in both deciduous and permanent dentitions. In fusion the tooth count is one less when compared to gemination. Fusion can occur between two normal tooth germs or between a normal and a supernumerary tooth; radiographically two separate pulp chambers can be appreciated [37].

Studies have reported hereditary, genetic, and environmental factors responsible for gemination and fusion. The treatment approach is usually multidisciplinary depending on the teeth involved, patient requirement, and degree of involvement [37, 38].

- **Concrescence**

Concrescence is defined as the fusion of two fully formed adjacent teeth along the root surface by cementum only without the confluence of the underlying dentin [39]. It is usually an asymptomatic condition and commonly seen in the region of the maxillary molars. Theories suggest the lack of interdental bone and periodontal ligament stimulus as factors responsible for the fusion of the appositional cemental layers between the roots of adjacent teeth [40]. Concrescence is best evaluated radiographically, and therefore preoperative radiographs should be considered during third molar extractions to avoid surgical complications and during orthodontic treatments [41].

- **Dilaceration**

Dilaceration is defined as the change in the axial inclination of the crown of a tooth to its root or a sharp bend or curve in the crown or root of a formed tooth [42]. The most acceptable cause is mechanical trauma to the primary predecessor tooth, although several other factors such as ectopic development of the tooth germ, extraction of deciduous tooth roots, and hereditary factors have been implicated [42]. Dilaceration can be seen in both primary and permanent dentitions, unilaterally or bilaterally with an incidence ranging from 0.32% to 98% [43]. Although dilaceration in the crown can be diagnosed clinically for root dilacerations, preoperative panoramic radiographs are mandatory prior to performing endodontic treatment, extraction, and orthodontic treatment [44].

- **Talon's Cusp**

Talon's cusp is an accessory cusp that projects from the palatal or lingual surfaces of the maxillary and mandibular permanent incisors in the shape of a three-pronged pattern resembling an eagle's talon [45]. It is composed of enamel and dentin but may or may not consist of pulpal tissue. There may be the presence of a developmental groove where the cusp fuses with the lingual surface of the tooth. Talon's cusp is frequently seen in the permanent dentition, although a few cases in the deciduous dentition have been reported [46]. It occurs either unilaterally or bilaterally with a predilection for the maxilla than the mandible. It is most seen in association with maxillary lateral incisors (67%), followed by central incisors (24%) and canines (9%) [47]. Studies have reported a multifactorial etiology that includes hyperactivity of the enamel organ during morphodifferentiation and genetic and hereditary factors [45]. Talon's cusp is associated with syndromes such as the Rubinstein-Taybi syndrome and Sturge-Weber syndrome [48]. The presence of a talon's cusp can lead to carious developmental grooves, occlusal interference, periodontal problems, aesthetic concerns, and speech, mastication, and nursing difficulties. It may also remain dormant causing no discomfort [49]. Treatment modalities such as periodic observations, aesthetic restorations, application of topical fluorides and sealants, and root canal treatments should be considered for the aforementioned problems [50].

- **Dens Invaginatus**

Dens invaginatus (DI) also termed as "dens in dente" is a developmental anomaly which is the result of an invagination in the surface of the tooth crown before calcification or radicular invagination resulting from an infolding of Hertwig's epithelial root sheath [51]. The permanent maxillary lateral incisors are the most frequently involved tooth which is usually bilaterally. According to several studies, Oehler's classification of DI is the most widely accepted; Class I is a partial invagination that is confined to the crown of the tooth. These lesions involve dentine and enamel but do not extend past the cementoenamel junction (CEJ) or involve the pulp. Class II is a partial invagination that extends beyond the crown of the tooth and into the root, beyond the CEJ. These lesions may or may not involve pulp but remain within the anatomy of the root. There is no communication with the periodontal ligament. Class IIIa is the complete invagination which extends through the root. It communicates with the periodontal ligament through a second foramen on the lateral aspect of the tooth. There is usually no involvement of the pulp itself, but it causes a significant anatomical malformation. Class IIIb is the complete invagination that extends through the root and communicates with the periodontal ligament at the apical foramen. Again, often there is no direct involvement of the pulpal anatomy, but the lesion causes significant disruption to the dental anatomy [52, 53]. Radiographic evaluation is a must for diagnosis of DI, and one can observe a "pear-shaped" invagination of enamel and dentin. Cone-beam computed tomography (CBCT) is preferred to assess DI prior to treatment. Teeth with DI exhibit susceptibility to dental caries, pulpal necrosis, and periapical pathologies. A wide range of prophylactic treatment options such as preventive resin restorations, root canal treatment, and apexification should be considered depending upon the clinical situation [54].

- **Dens Evaginatus**

Dens evaginatus (DE) also referred to as "Leong's premolar" is a developmental anomaly that clinically appears as a cusp-like elevation or globule of enamel located on the occlusal surfaces between the buccal and lingual cusps of premolars or molars and the palatal and lingual surfaces of anterior teeth, either unilaterally or bilaterally [51]. In accordance with the available literature till date, there are two types of DE, a hornlike projection on the lingual or palatal surfaces of the anterior teeth referred to as "talon's cusp" or enamel tubercle on the occlusal surfaces of the posterior teeth predominantly the premolars [51]. DE is prevalent among the Asian population with an incidence of 0.5–4.3% [55, 56]. The etiology concerning DE has been explained to occur during the morphodifferentiation stage of odontogenesis, where there is an abnormal proliferation of the inner enamel epithelium and the ectomesenchymal layer of the dental papilla (subjacent ectomesenchyme) into the stellate reticulum. With the presence of such dental anomalies, individuals encounter the risk of occlusal wear or fracture leading to pulpal pathosis and may contribute to delayed eruption. Treatment modalities could range from root canal treatments to aesthetic and conservative approaches such as enameloplasty or tubercle grinding [51].

- **Taurodontism**

Taurodontism is a dental anomaly in which the body of the tooth is enlarged at the expense of the roots resembling the tooth of a cud-chewing animal, hence also called as "bull-like" teeth caused by the delay or failure of Hertwig's epithelial root sheath to invaginate at a proper horizontal level [57]. Taurodontism is predominantly seen in the permanent dentition affecting the molars either unilaterally or bilaterally with no gender predilection and an incidence ranging from 0.5% to 46% [57]. Studies have reported an association of taurodontism with several syndromes such as amelogenesis imperfecta, cleft lip and palate, Down syndrome, ectodermal dysplasia, Klinefelter's syndrome, and osteogenesis imperfecta [58]. Taurodontism was classified by Shaw in 1928 based on the displacement of the floor of the pulpal chamber at the expense of the roots. There are four types: cynodont (normal), hypotaurodontism (teeth with slightly enlarged pulp chambers), mesotaurodontism (teeth with much enlarged pulp chambers with shorter roots), and hypertaurodontism (pulp chambers that nearly reach the apex of the roots) [57]. Treatment modalities such as root canal treatment, extractions, and orthodontic procedures can be challenging due to the susceptibility of the tooth to root resorption, anchorage value, and the apical placement of the pulp chambers. Successful diagnosis and treatment would largely depend upon appropriate imaging techniques. Recent studies have emphasized the use of cone-beam computed tomography for better clarity, reliability, and 3D constructs when compared to panoramic radiographs.

2.7.4 *Developmental Disturbances in Structure of Teeth*

- **Amelogenesis Imperfecta**

Amelogenesis imperfecta (AI) is a group of hereditary disorders affecting the structure and appearance of dental enamel [59]. Amelogenesis process, formation, and maturation of dental enamel are controlled by specialized epithelial-derived cells, ameloblasts, which secrete extracellular matrix containing different types of extracellular matrix proteins including mainly amelogenin, enamelin, ameloblastin, and amelotin. In addition to extracellular matrix proteins, ameloblast secretes matrix enzymes such as kallikrein-4 and matrix metalloproteinaise-20 [59]. The prevalence of AI ranges from 1:700 to 1:14,000 affecting almost all the teeth of the primary and secondary dentition [60]. Mutations in several genes such as amelogenin gene (AMELX) and enamelin gene (ENAM), among others, have been implicated in the pathogenesis of different forms of AI. The clinical phenotype and the mode of inheritance were the basic principles that have been used to classify AI for the last century [59].

Clinically, AI was classified into three main groups: hypoplastic, hypocalcified, and hypomaturation types.

Hypoplastic AI usually reflects a defect during the secretory stage of the ameloblast as during this stage, matrix is laid down and the crystals grow in length, thereby defining the enamel thickness. Hypoplastic enamel defects can be classified as generalized, localized, or pitted [59].

The hypocalcified AI type is distinguished by enamel that is so poorly mineralized that it can be scraped away easily and fails very rapidly. Hypocalcified AI usually results from a defect in the crystal initiation during the enamel formation [59].

Hypomaturation AI is characterized by weak, opaque, and discolored enamel that lacks normal translucency and inappropriately retains enamel matrix proteins. Hypomaturation AI is usually considered to result from a defect during the maturation stage where the degraded enamel matrix protein should be removed [59].

Patients diagnosed with AI encounter psychological and functional concerns. A multidisciplinary and conservative approach is best suggested for AI. Studies have suggested a full-mouth prosthetic treatment as the best treatment modality for patients with AI.

- **Dentinogenesis Imperfecta**

Dentinogenesis imperfecta (DI) is an autosomal dominant disorder of the dentin affecting both primary and permanent dentitions, caused due to the mutation in the dentin sialophosphoprotein (DSPP) [61]. DI can have different types including the following: type I is DI with osteogenesis imperfecta (OI), type II is DI without OI, and type III is brandywine type characterized by shell teeth, with very little dentin and multiple pulp exposure in the primary teeth. Clinically, in both DI type I and type II, the affected teeth are yellowish to blue gray or amber brown in color with an opalescent and translucent hue. Radiographically, the affected teeth have bulbous crowns, narrow or constricted roots, and pulp chambers which are either smaller than the normal or completely obliterated [62].

The management aspect for patients diagnosed with DI varies depending upon the type of dentition involved and the severity of the condition. It largely focuses on eliminating the source of infection, restoring aesthetics, and protecting the posterior teeth. For primary dentition, composite strip crowns for anterior teeth and stainless-steel crowns for posterior teeth can be used to prevent tooth wear. For permanent dentition, intervention should be considered only if required. Treatment modalities could range from restorations, full-mouth rehabilitation, dental implants, and endodontic therapies followed by routine dental checkups [63].

- **Dentin Dysplasia**

Dentin dysplasia (DD) is also referred to as "rootless teeth." It is a rare autosomal dominant defect characterized by atypical dentin formation affecting both primary and permanent dentitions [64]. DD is classified as DD type 1 (radicular dentin dysplasia) and DD type 2 (coronal dentin dysplasia), with a higher prevalence rate (1 in every 100,000) of DD type 1. In DD type 1, the affected teeth rarely appear amber colored [62]. They exhibit increased tooth mobility and exfoliate prematurely. Radiographically, the pulp chamber and root canals are obliterated in the deciduous dentition, whereas remnants of the pulpal tissue are seen in the permanent dentition. The roots are short blunted and conical in both deciduous and permanent dentitions. In DD type 2, the deciduous teeth appear yellow to brown to bluish gray in color, whereas the permanent teeth appear normal clinically [64]. Radiographically, permanent teeth have enlarged pulp chambers with a "thistle tube" configuration. DD type 1 is associated with periapical radiolucencies such as cysts, granulomas, and abscesses. The treatment aspect for patients with DD is challenging as it involves restorative, endodontic, and prosthetic approaches. Recent studies have shown successful results with the placement of dental implants to restore aesthetics and functionality for patients.

- **Regional Odontodysplasia**

Regional odontodysplasia (RO) also referred to as "ghost teeth" is a rare nonhereditary dental anomaly characterized by hypoplastic and hypocalcified enamel and dentin [65]. Although there is no definitive etiology, a few factors such as trauma, latent virus infection, circulatory disorders, radiation, and nutritional deficiencies have been reported as plausible factors for RO. It is known to affect both deciduous and permanent dentitions in a localized pattern with female predominance (1.4:1) than males. It also affects the maxilla twice (66%) as the mandible and exhibits a tendency of affecting only one quadrant. Clinically, the affected teeth are irregular in appearance with yellowish brown discoloration. The most common observation radiographically is the "ghost teeth"-like appearance due to the presence of extremely thin enamel and dentin with large radiolucent pulp chambers. The most accepted treatment modality is the extraction of the affected tooth followed by prosthetic replacements using dental implants to restore both aesthetic and functional elements of the dentition.

2.8 Conclusion

A proper interpretation of the normal as well as the abnormal dental anatomy may make the difference in the decision-making. Different radiographs are generating 2D images for both dental arches. They are considered the main routinely used diagnostic tools for overviewing dental condition of the patient. However, it has main pitfalls and limitations related to its two-dimensional nature, such as overlapping of anatomic structures and distortion. Artificial intelligence (AI)-based methods can help dentists to interpret images in an automated way which may enable faster identification and classification of data and eliminate errors associated with human. A study was conducted by Hiraiwa et al., in 2019, in which panoramic radiographs for 400 patients (50% male and 50% female) were used for training convolutional neural networks (CNNs) which is a subtype of deep learning machines [66]. The study aimed to identify the morphology and the number of the distal root of 760 mandibular first molars using deep learning machines and compared to the gold standard CBCT findings. The study found that CBCT images showed 21.4% of distal roots have an extra roots for the mandibular first molar. Moreover, the study demonstrated that the diagnostic accuracy of deep learning was 86.9% for the determination of the number of distal roots whether it was a simple root or having extra roots that was higher than expert radiologists [66].

Another recent study conducted by Lee et al., in 2022, used 22,999 panoramic dental images to train faster R-CNN models, a type of deep learning machines, trying to detect 17 dental anomalies including calcifications, caries, and anomalies in dental and surrounding dental regions [67]. In this study, seven dental anomalies were targeted to be detected by convolutional neural network model including supernumerary tooth, periapical radiolucency, residual root, external root absorption, and impacted tooth. The study showed that CNNs succeeded to identify the mentioned anomalies with different specificity but in general very high accuracy. For example, automatic identification of supernumerary teeth was 97.4%, external root resorption 99.3%, impacted teeth 92.3%, periapical radiolucency 89.5%, residual root 97.2%, and tooth overlapped with mandibular canal 93.4% [67].

Most of the abovementioned dental anomalies cause aesthetic and functional problems. In most of cases, different treatment modalities can be required ranging from orthodontic treatment to restorative treatments (composite or porcelain veneers), endodontic treatment, or sometimes surgical extractions depending upon each case scenario [25].

References

1. Ash MM (1993) Wheeler's dental anatomy, physiology, and occlusion. W.B. Saunders, Philadelphia. https://www.elsevier.com/books/wheelers-dental-anatomy-physiology-and-occlusion/nelson/978-0-323-63878-4
2. Physiologic tooth movement: eruption and shedding. In: Ten Cate's oral histology. Elsevier, Amsterdam, pp 233–252 (2013)

3. Dental numbering system-primary teeth. http://www.americantooth.com/downloads/instructions/Dental_Sys_Primary_Teeth.pdf
4. Dental numbering system permanent teeth. http://www.americantooth.com/downloads/instructions/Dental_Sys_Permanent_Teeth.pdf
5. Pocket dentistry-introduction to dental anatomy. https://pocketdentistry.com/1-introduction-to-dental-anatomy/
6. Morris AL, Tadi P (2022 Jan) Anatomy, head and neck, teeth. [Updated 2021 July 31]. In: StatPearls [Internet]. StatPearls Publishing, Treasure Island. Available from: https://www.ncbi.nlm.nih.gov/books/NBK557543/
7. Zajac JC, Abbate O, Oh AK, Mantilla-Rivas E, Aivaz M, Wang R, Talbet J, Manrique M, Tate AR, Rogers GF (2020 June) Dental topics for plastic surgeons, part one: normal anatomy, growth and development. J Craniofac Surg 31(4):1168–1173. https://doi.org/10.1097/SCS.0000000000006370
8. Introductory chapter: the importance of gingival treatment and prevention. Scientific figure on ResearchGate. Available from: https://www.researchgate.net/figure/The-periodontium-components_fig3_332391780. Accessed 22 Apr 2022
9. Thesleff I (2003) Epithelial-mesenchymal signalling regulating tooth morphogenesis. J Cell Sci 116(Pt 9):1647–1648. https://doi.org/10.1242/jcs.00410
10. Kwon HE, Jia S, Lan Y, Liu H, Jiang R (2017) Activin and Bmp4 signaling converge on Wnt activation during odontogenesis. J Dent Res 96(10):1145–1152. https://doi.org/10.1177/0022034517713710
11. Tompkins K (2006) Molecular mechanisms of cytodifferentiation in mammalian tooth development. Connect Tissue Res 47(3):111–118. https://doi.org/10.1080/03008200600727756
12. Bei M (2009) Molecular genetics of tooth development. Curr Opin Genet Dev 19(5):504–510. https://doi.org/10.1016/j.gde.2009.09.002
13. Lee JM, Qin C, Chai OH, Lan Y, Jiang R, Kwon HE (2022) MSX1 drives tooth morphogenesis through controlling Wnt signaling activity. J Dent Res:220345211070583. https://doi.org/10.1177/00220345211070583
14. Thesleff I, Tummers M (2008) Tooth organogenesis and regeneration *StemBook*. Harvard Stem Cell Institute, Cambridge, MA
15. Bilgir E, Bayrakdar İŞ, Çelik Ö, Orhan K, Akkoca F, Sağlam H et al (2021) An artificial ıntelligence approach to automatic tooth detection and numbering in panoramic radiographs. BMC Med Imaging 21(1):1–9
16. Lin P-L, Lai Y-H, Huang P-W (2010) An effective classification and numbering system for dental bitewing radiographs using teeth region and contour information. Pattern Recogn 43(4):1380–1392
17. Chen Y, Zhou F, Peng Y, Chen L, Wang Y (2019) Non-syndromic occurrence of true generalized microdontia with hypodontia: a case report. Medicine 98(26):e16283. https://doi.org/10.1097/MD.0000000000016283
18. Tuzoff DV, Tuzova LN, Bornstein MM, Krasnov AS, Kharchenko MA, Nikolenko SI et al (2019) Tooth detection and numbering in panoramic radiographs using convolutional neural networks. Dentomaxillofac Radiol 48(4):20180051
19. McKinney R, Olmo H (2022) Developmental disturbances of the teeth, anomalies of shape and size *StatPearls*. StatPearls Publishing, Treasure Island
20. Bargale SD, Kiran SDP (2011) Non-syndromic occurrence of true generalized microdontia with mandibular mesiodens - a rare case. Head Face Med 7(1):19. https://doi.org/10.1186/1746-160X-7-19
21. Fekonja A (2017) Prevalence of dental developmental anomalies of permanent teeth in children and their influence on esthetics. J Esthet Restor Dent 29(4):276–283. https://doi.org/10.1111/jerd.12302
22. Chetty M, Beshtawi K, Roomaney I, Kabbashi S (2021) MACRODONTIA: a brief overview and a case report of KBG syndrome. Radiol Case Rep 16(6):1305–1310. https://doi.org/10.1016/j.radcr.2021.02.068

23. Mainali A, Denny C, Sumanth K, Ongole R (2010) Non syndromic generalised macrodontia. J Nepal Dent Assoc 11(2):150–153
24. Canoglu E, Canoglu H, Aktas A, Cehreli ZC (2012) Isolated bilateral macrodontia of mandibular second premolars: a case report. Eur J Dent 6(3):330–334
25. Laverty DP, Thomas MBM (2016) The restorative management of microdontia. Br Dent J 221(4):160–166. https://doi.org/10.1038/sj.bdj.2016.595
26. Al-Ani AH, Antoun JS, Thomson WM, Merriman TR, Farella M (2017) Hypodontia: an update on its etiology, classification, and clinical management. BioMed Res Int 2017:9378325
27. Kaushal K, Kim E-J, Tyagi A, Karapurkar JK, Haq S, Jung H-S et al (2022) Genome-wide screening for deubiquitinase subfamily identifies ubiquitin-specific protease 49 as a novel regulator of odontogenesis. Cell Death Differ 29:1–16
28. Rajab L, Hamdan M (2002) Supernumerary teeth: review of the literature and a survey of 152 cases. Int J Paediatr Dent 12(4):244–254
29. Lu X, Yu F, Liu J, Cai W, Zhao Y, Zhao S, Liu S (2017) The epidemiology of supernumerary teeth and the associated molecular mechanism. Organogenesis 13(3):71–82
30. Lubinsky M, Kantaputra PN (2016) Syndromes with supernumerary teeth. Am J Med Genet A 170(10):2611–2616
31. Mhaske S, Yuwanati MB, Mhaske A, Ragavendra R, Kamath K, Saawarn S (2013) Natal and neonatal teeth: an overview of the literature. ISRN Pediatr 2013:956269
32. Shivpuri A, Mitra R, Saxena V, Shivpuri A (2021) Natal and neonatal teeth: clinically relevant findings in a retrospective analysis. Med J Armed Forces India 77(2):154–157
33. Cunha RF, Boer FAC, Torriani DD, Frossard WTG (2001) Natal and neonatal teeth: review of the literature. Pediatr Dent 23(2):158–162
34. Jamani NA, Ardini YD, Harun NA (2018) Neonatal tooth with Riga-fide disease affecting breastfeeding: a case report. Int Breastfeed J 13(1):1–4
35. Bulut G, Bulut H, Ortac R (2019) A comprehensive survey of natal and neonatal teeth in newborns. Niger J Clin Pract 22(11):1489–1489
36. Ben Salem M, Chouchene F, Masmoudi F, Baaziz A, Maatouk F, Ghedira H (2021) Fusion or gemination? Diagnosis and management in primary teeth: A report of two cases. Case Rep Dent 2021(1):1–6
37. Sekerci AE, Sisman Y, Yasa Y, Sahman H, Ekizer A (2011) Prevalence of fusion and gemination in permanent teeth in Cappadocia region in Turkey. Pak Oral Dent J 31(1):15–20
38. Venkatesh A, Mitthra S, Prakash V, Prasad TS (2016) Gemination or fusion? – a case report. Biomed Pharmacol J 9(3):1225–1228
39. Gernhofer KJ (2009) Concrescence of a maxillary second and third molar. J Calif Dent Assoc 37(7):479–481
40. Peterkova R, Peterka M, Viriot L, Lesot H (2000) Dentition development and budding morphogenesis. J Craniofac Genet Dev Biol 20(4):158–172
41. Consolaro A, Hadaya O, Miranda DAO, Consolaro RB (2020) Concrescence: can the teeth involved be moved or separated? Dent Press J Orthod 25:20–25
42. Topouzelis N, Tsaousoglou P, Pisoka V, Zouloumis L (2010) Dilaceration of maxillary central incisor: a literature review. Dent Traumatol 26(5):427–433
43. Hamasha A, Al-Khateeb T, Darwazeh A (2002) Prevalence of dilaceration in Jordanian adults. Int Endod J 35(11):910–912
44. Jafarzadeh H, Abbott PV (2007) Dilaceration: review of an endodontic challenge. J Endod 33(9):1025–1030
45. Tulunoglu O, Cankala D, Ozdemir R (2007) Talon's cusp: report of four unusual cases. J Indian Soc Pedod Prev Dent 25(1):52
46. Sarpangala M, Devasya A (2017) Variants of talon cusp (dens evaginatus). J Clin Diagn Res 11(1):ZJ01
47. Bahadure RN, Thosar N, Jain ES (2012) Management of talons cusp associated with primary central incisor: a rare case report. Int J Clin Pediatr Dent 5(2):142
48. Dunn WJ (2004) Unusual case of labial and lingual talon cusps. Mil Med 169(2):108–110

49. Hattab FN, Yassin OM, Al-Nimri KS (1995) Talon cusp-clinical significance and management. Quintessence Int Engl Ed 26:115–115
50. Gupta R, Thakur N, Thakur S, Gupta B, Gupta M (2013) Talon cusp: a case report with management guidelines for practicing dentists. Dent Hypotheses 4(2):67
51. Mupparapu M, Singer S, Goodchild J (2004) Dens evaginatus and dens invaginatus in a maxillary lateral incisor: report of a rare occurrence and review of literature. Aust Dent J 49(4):201–203
52. Gündüz K, Çelenk P, Canger EM, Zengin Z, Sümer P (2013) A retrospective study of the prevalence and characteristics of dens invaginatus in a sample of the Turkish population. Med Oral Patol Oral Cirugía Bucal 18(1):e27
53. Oehlers F (1958) The radicular variety of dens invaginatus. Oral Surg Oral Med Oral Pathol 11(11):1251–1260
54. Azzahim L, Bassim N, Abdallaoui F (2022) CBCT evaluation and conservative management of a large periapical lesion associated with dens invaginatus type II. Case Rep Dent 2022:1529835
55. Cho S, Ki Y, Chu V, Chan J (2006) Concomitant developmental dental anomalies in Chinese children with dens evaginatus. Int J Paediatr Dent 16(4):247–251
56. Lin C-S, Llacer-Martinez M, Sheth CC, Jovani-Sancho M, Biedma BM (2018) Prevalence of premolars with dens evaginatus in a Taiwanese and Spanish population and related complications of the fracture of its tubercle. Eur Endod J 3(2):118
57. Dineshshankar J, Sivakumar M, Balasubramanium AM, Kesavan G, Karthikeyan M, Prasad VS (2014) Taurodontism. J Pharm Bioallied Sci 6(Suppl 1):S13
58. Manjunatha B, Kovvuru SK (2010) Taurodontism: a review on its etiology, prevalence, and clinical considerations. J Clin Exp Dent 2(4):1–5
59. Smith CE, Poulter JA, Antanaviciute A, Kirkham J, Brookes SJ, Inglehearn CF, Mighell AJ (2017) Amelogenesis imperfecta; genes, proteins, and pathways. Front Physiol 435. https://doi.org/10.3389/fphys.2017.00435
60. Crawford PJ, Aldred M, Bloch-Zupan A (2007) Amelogenesis imperfecta. Orphanet J Rare Dis 2(1):1–11
61. Majorana A, Bardellini E, Brunelli PC, Lacaita M, Cazzolla AP, Favia G (2010) Dentinogenesis imperfecta in children with osteogenesis imperfecta: a clinical and ultrastructural study. Int J Paediatr Dent 20(2):112–118
62. de La Dure-Molla M, Philippe Fournier B, Berdal A (2015) Isolated dentinogenesis imperfecta and dentin dysplasia: revision of the classification. Eur J Hum Genet 23(4):445–451
63. Barron MJ, McDonnell ST, MacKie I, Dixon MJ (2008) Hereditary dentine disorders: dentinogenesis imperfecta and dentine dysplasia. Orphanet J Rare Dis 3(1):1–10
64. Toomarian L, Mashhadiabbas F, Mirkarimi M, Mehrdad L (2010) Dentin dysplasia type I: a case report and review of the literature. J Med Case Rep 4(1):1–6
65. Hamdan MA, Sawair FA, Rajab LD, Hamdan AM, Al-Omari IK (2004) Regional odontodysplasia: a review of the literature and report of a case. Int J Paediatr Dent 14(5):363–370
66. Hiraiwa T, Ariji Y, Fukuda M, Kise Y, Nakata K, Katsumata A et al (2019) A deep-learning artificial intelligence system for assessment of root morphology of the mandibular first molar on panoramic radiography. Dentomaxillofac Radiol 48(3):20180218
67. Lee S, Kim D, Jeong H-G (2022) Detecting 17 fine-grained dental anomalies from panoramic dental radiography using artificial intelligence. Sci Rep 12(1):5172. https://doi.org/10.1038/s41598-022-09083-2

Chapter 3
Most Common Oral Health Conditions

Oral diseases are one of the most common diseases that affect human beings. It can exist as a primary cause of a disease such as dental caries, periodontal diseases, oral mucosal lesions, and premalignant and malignant conditions. In addition, oral diseases can occur as secondary to different and several systemic conditions such as diabetes mellitus, HIV infection, and drug administration. Recently and realizing the importance of oral health, it has been a call for incorporating oral health status in overall health-care diagnosis after a long time of dealing with oral health as a separate condition [1].

Recently, different artificial intelligence-based technologies such as deep learning, convolutional neural network, and artificial intelligence-based algorithms have been used to identify, classify, diagnose, and predict prognosis and treatment outcomes of most of oral health conditions [2, 3]. AI has been used to investigate dental caries, periodontal diseases, oral cancers, Sjögren's syndrome, oral lesions, oral clefts, etc. The results of implementation of AI in detection, diagnosis and classification of oral health conditions are extremely promising.

3.1 Prevalence of Oral Disease

Globally, it is estimated that 2.3 billion people suffer from caries of permanent teeth, and more than 530 million children suffer from caries of primary teeth. Dental caries or tooth decay is the most common oral disease, and according to this study (1900–2010), the untreated tooth decay ranks 36th as the most prevalent oral disease among 291 different conditions [5]. In addition and according to the same report, severe tooth loss affects an estimated 2% of the global population. According to the World Health Organization (WHO) published in April 2012, 30% of people ages 65–74 years have lost all of their natural teeth that have great impact on their quality of life. The variability and inconsistency about the prevalence of oral disease

K. Shaikh et al., *Artificial Intelligence in Dentistry*,
https://doi.org/10.1007/978-3-031-19715-4_3

may be attributing to the difference and variability of wealth, living conditions, health-care accessibility, and educational attainments of these population and countries. For example, one study found that the data collected from 20 countries from Eastern Mediterranean Region (EMRO) showed that the prevalence of the dental caries among 12 years is higher in the primary teeth than the permanent dentition [6].

In most low- and middle-income countries, with increasing urbanization and changes in living conditions, the prevalence of oral diseases continues to increase. This is primarily due to inadequate exposure to fluoride (in the water supply and oral hygiene products such as toothpaste) and poor access to oral health-care services in the community. Marketing of food and beverages high in sugar, as well as tobacco and alcohol, has led to a growing consumption of products that contribute to oral health conditions and other noncommunicable diseases [4].

The adverse effects of inadequate care for teeth, gums, bite, and jaws can move beyond the mouth to affect overall physical and psychological health. Research has indicated that poor oral health may be associated with medical conditions such as heart disease, stroke, diabetes, pneumonia, and other respiratory diseases. It has also been linked to preterm births and low-birth-weight babies. Jaw problems are also a common cause of headaches and ear and facial pain. Dental clearance prior to medical treatment, including cancer/bisphosphonate therapy and cardiac surgery, minimizes both oral and systemic complications. Many medical conditions have oral manifestations, and some medications have side effects that lead to compromised oral health as well as jaw function disabilities [7].

In collaboration with medical and allied health professionals, dental specialists also manage a variety of medically related problems, including oral/jaw pathologies, orofacial traumas, head and neck tumors, obstructive sleep apnea, and temporomandibular disorder-related (TMD) headaches and ear problems [8].

3.2 Most Common Dental Diseases

Oral conditions like dental caries and periodontal (gum) disease continue to plague humanity since time immemorial. Other predominant oral health conditions are oral cancers, oral manifestations of HIV, oro-dental trauma, cleft lip and palate, and Noma (severe gangrenous disease starting in the mouth mostly affecting children). Most oral health conditions are largely preventable and can be treated in their early stages.

The *Global Burden of Disease Study 2017* estimated that oral diseases affect close to 3.5 billion people worldwide, with caries of permanent teeth being the most common condition [4].

3.2.1 Dental Caries (Tooth Decay)

Dental caries result when plaque forms on the surface of a tooth and converts the free sugars (all sugars added to foods by the manufacturer, cook, or consumer, plus sugars naturally present in honey, syrups, and fruit juices) contained in foods and drinks into acids that destroy the tooth over time. A continued high intake of free sugars, inadequate exposure to fluoride, and a lack of removal of plaque by tooth brushing can lead to caries, pain, and sometimes tooth loss and infection [4].

According to **Shafer**, **Hine**, and **Levy**, dental caries is an irreversible microbial disease of the calcified tissues of the teeth, characterized by demineralization of the inorganic portion and destruction of the organic substance of the tooth, which often leads to cavitations. The word caries is derived from the Latin word meaning "rot" or "decay." It is a complex and dynamic process where a multitude of factors initiate and influence the progression of disease. Although effective methods are known for prevention and management of dental caries, it is a major health problem with manifestations persisting throughout life despite treatment. It is seen in all geographic areas in the world and affects persons of both genders in all races, all socioeconomic strata, and every age group. Some stay "caries-free" for unknown reason [9].

- **Epidemiology**

Caries was referred to as "a disease of civilization." Prehistoric man had decreased prevalence of dental caries. Decreased caries prevalence is seen in African and Asian communities also [10].

Factors Affecting Caries Prevalence

- **Race**—Some evidence indicates that blacks, Chinese, and East Indians have considerably less caries than American Whites. The English have a higher caries incidence than Italians, Russians, and Chinese.
- **Age**—Children from families in lower socioeconomic groups consistently have greater caries prevalence than their peers from families at a higher socioeconomic level.
- **Sex**—The total caries experience in permanent teeth is greater in females than in males of the same age. This is attributable largely to the fact that the teeth of girls erupt at an earlier age.
- **Familial**—Siblings of individuals with high caries susceptibility are also generally caries active, whereas siblings of caries immune individuals generally exhibit low caries rates. Children of parents with a low caries experience also tend to have low caries; the converse is true for children whose parents have a high caries rate [9].

- **Etiology of Dental Caries**

Dental caries etiology has four main factors: bacteria, time, susceptible tooth surface, and fermentable carbohydrates (Fig. 3.1).

The etiology of dental caries is generally agreed to be a complex problem complicated by many indirect factors that obscure the direct cause or causes. There is no

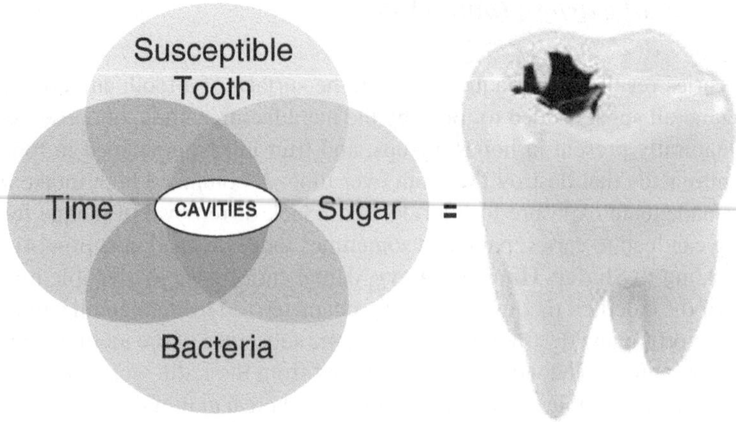

Fig. 3.1 Factors causing dental caries

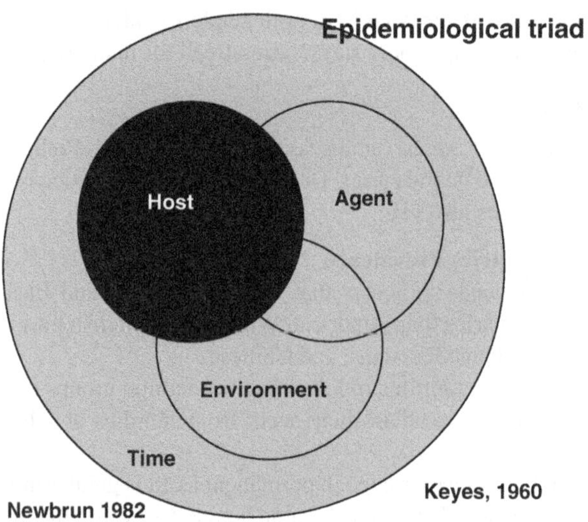

Fig. 3.2 Newbrun Tetralogy

universally accepted opinion for the etiology of dental caries. Numerous references on dental caries, including early theories attempting to explain its etiology, have been found in recorded history of ancient people. However, many theories have evolved through years of investigation and observation; the acidogenic theory of Miller (Miller's chemico-parasitic theory), the proteolytic theory, and the proteolysis-chelation theory, are among those which have stood the test of time [9, 11–13] (Fig. 3.2).

- **Current Concepts of Caries Etiology**

Dental caries is a multifactorial disease with interplay of three primary factors: the host, the microbial flora, and the substrate as put forward by Keyes in 1960. Later in 1982, Newbrun included time as an inevitable fourth factor. In other words, caries requires a susceptible host, a cariogenic flora, and a suitable substrate that must be present for a sufficient length of time. Conversely, caries prevention is based upon attempts to increase the resistance of the host, lower the number of microorganisms in contact with the tooth, and modify the substrate by selecting non-cariogenic foodstuffs and reduce the time that the substrate is in the mouth [9].

- **Contributing Factors in Dental Caries**

The mere presence of microorganisms and a suitable substrate at a given point on a tooth surface is insufficient to establish a carious lesion in all individuals. Variations in caries incidence are due to the presence of a number of indirect or contributing factors.

A workshop on dental caries mechanisms and control techniques was held at the University of Michigan in 1947. This group listed a number of indirect factors that might influence the etiology of caries [9] (Table 3.1).

- **Clinical Classification of Caries [9, 14]**

1. Sturdevant
   (a) Based on: a. Location
      – Primary
      – Caries of pit and fissure origin

Table 3.1 Factors that influence in caries etiology

Host factors	Components
Tooth	1. Composition 2. Morphologic characteristics 3. Position
Saliva	1. Composition a) Inorganic b) Organic 2. pH 3. Quantity 4. Viscosity 5. Antibacterial factors
Diet	1. Physical factors a) Quality of diet 2. Local factors a) Carbohydrate content b) Vitamin content c) Fluorine content
Systemic conditions	

Image source: Shafer's Textbook of Oral Pathology [9]

  - Caries of enamel smooth surface origin
  - Backward caries
  - Forward caries
  - Residual caries
  - Root surface caries
  - Secondary (recurrent) caries

(b) Extent

  - Incipient (reversible)
  - Cavitated (irreversible)

(c) Rate of progression

  - Acute (rampant)
  - Chronic (slow or arrested)

2. G.V Black [15] (Table 3.2)

- **Relevance of Early Detection of Dental Caries**

Globally, dental caries is still considered one of the most common chronic diseases that causes a major global health burden [16]. According to the latest epidemiology statistics, untreated dental caries in permanent teeth represents 65.71% of oral disorders. The sequelae of untreated caries can be transient causing reversible pulpitis or can be more permanent causing irreversible pulpitis, pulp necrosis,

Table 3.2 G. V Black classification of caries

Description	Classes	Illustration
Class I: Caries affecting pits and fissures on occlusal third of molars and premolars, occlusal two-thirds of molars and premolars, and lingual part of anterior teeth.	Class I	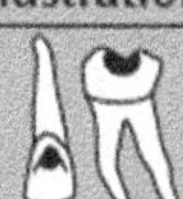
Class II: Caries affecting proximal surfaces of molars and premolars.	Class II	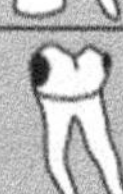
Class III: Caries affecting proximal surfaces of central incisors, lateral incisors, and cuspids without involving the incisal angles.	Class III	
Class IV: Caries affecting proximal including incisal angles of anterior teeth.	Class IV	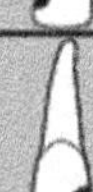
Class V: Caries affecting gingival one-third of facial or lingual surfaces of anterior or posterior teeth.	Class V	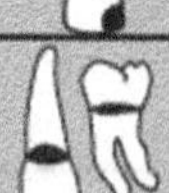
Class VI: Caries affecting cusp tips of molars, premolars, and cuspids	Class VI	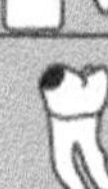

periapical abscess, and eventually tooth loss. Recording the dental status is one of the recurring and routinely tasks in dentistry during which a dentist is trying to detect and diagnose the pathological findings, including dental caries. The idea of this evaluation and assessment is to enable the dentist eventually to customize a preventive and treatment operative plan [17].

Visual examination (VE) including clinical examination where dentists usually use dental probe is the preferred clinical method for assessing and diagnosing dental caries, as it can be performed easily and achieve acceptable accuracy [18]. In this method, dentists rely on their observation to determine whether the tooth has carious lesion or not; in addition, dentist can use different types of radiographs to help for proper diagnosis.

Nevertheless, some studies showed that VE can miss detection of certain types of caries such as proximal caries, for example, it was found that the bitewing radiography has a low sensitivity. In addition, the literature is full of studies that reported and confirmed poor diagnostic sensitivity for detection of enamel demineralization by using regular radiographic images [19]. Furthermore, it has been observed that there are sometimes discrepancy and variation in the diagnosis of dental caries by dentists in certain situations, even though diagnostic studies have demonstrated that well-trained dentists are generally able to achieve good intra- and inter-examiner reproducibility [20]. Therefore, the need for independent method of verification helps clinicians in decision-making which can enhance patient care. Artificial intelligence (AI)-based technology with its advantages can be the ideal tool to provide the desirable subjective analysis of the patient dental status [21].

Several studies were published recently using several AI-based technologies such as deep learning and convolutional neural networks (CNNs) and sometimes a combination of both to detect caries on dental x-rays [22, 23] or near-infrared light transillumination images [24]; in addition, other studies have used intraoral images for automatic, AI-based caries detection [25].

Using AI-based machine in detection of dental caries showed variable results. An early in vitro study using 160 radiographic images of extracted teeth to assess the presence of dental caries. The study showed that AI-based technology achieved diagnostic accuracy rate of 88.4% in comparison to 71.7% achieved by 25 examiners relying on their visual examination and clinical experiences. Hence, the study suggested that AI-based machines have improved the diagnoses of proximal caries detection by 39.4% in comparison to the one assessed visually by humans [26]. Another study showed that there is an increase in the sensitivity by 71% of the ability of dentists to detect enamel- only proximal caries by using AI software [27]. Another two studies showed that there is 80% accuracy of detection of dental carries using AI logarithms with respect to expert standards [28, 29] in addition to a study that was conducted by Sonavane et al., in 2021, using 74 visual images extracted from Kaggle dataset for teeth for training artificial neural network machine. The visual images were classified into 60 images for training purposes and 14 images for testing purposes. Furthermore, 45 images out of 60 were showing caries and the remaining 15 images having non-caries. The study demonstrated that using artificial neural network model was able to achieve 71.43% accuracy for classifying teeth into teeth with cavities and teeth without cavities [30].

However, a recent study published by Kuhnisch et al. aimed to develop a deep learning approach with convolutional neural networks (CNNs) for caries detection and to compare the diagnostic performance with respect to expert standards found that it was possible to achieve more than 90% agreement to detect caries and caries-related cavities using the AI method with standardized, single-tooth photographs. Nevertheless, the author suggested that using AI as an automated approach to detects caries needs further improvement [31]. Another recent study conducted by Zheng et al., in 2021, aimed to investigate the use of three different convolutional neural networks (CNNs) for detection of deep caries and pulpitis. The author integrates clinical parameters including chief complaint, pain history (spontaneous pain and location of pain), and clinical examination (deep cavity, probing and cold test) to CNNs to enhance and ensure best performance of CNNs to assess clinical diagnosis of deep caries and pulp pathosis [32]. The study showed that one of its CNN models achieved 82% accuracy, 81% precision, 85% sensitivity, and 82% specificity for detection of deep caries and pulpitis [32].

A recent study conducted by Javed et al., in 2020, investigated the possibility of using artificial neural network (ANN) to predict post-*Streptococcus mutans* prior to dental caries excavation that would help finally to have a caries-free cavity for final restoration [33]. The study demonstrated that using iOS app developed on artificial neural network (ANN) model succeeded in predicting post-*Streptococcus mutans* with an efficiency rate of 99%, which can help dentist to select the appropriate excavation method [33].

In order to investigate the cost-effectiveness of using conventional neural network (CNN) for accurate detection of proximal caries compared to bitewing radiographs, a recent study was conducted by Schwendicke et al., in 2021, who found that AI was able to detect caries with 80% accuracy rate, while dentist showed 71% [34]. Furthermore, sensitivity of AI was 75%, while for dentists was 36%, while AI specificity was not significantly lower than 83% versus 91% for dentist. Moreover, the study showed that AI was less costly and more effective for detection of dental caries [34].

Although using AI-based machines in detection of dental caries is showing promising results and expected to be more feasible in the future, there are some concerns and limitations about the potential use and application of the AI-based machines under clinical conditions, and they still recommend a need to be critically judged by professionals. The reason for this concern is the fact that to maintain perfect examination conditions in the daily dental practice cannot be maintained every time.

- **Diagnostic Aids in Dental Caries** [9, 35, 36]**:**

1. Visual inspection and tactile examination
2. Radiographs
3. Caries detecting dyes
4. Fiber-optic transillumination

5. Xeroradiography
6. Subtraction radiography
7. Mini-D
8. Fluorescence
   (a) QLF
   (b) DIAGNOdent
9. Carbon dioxide laser
10. Ultrasound caries detector
11. Endoscope/video scope
12. Micro-air abrasion
13. Tuned aperture computed tomography
14. Cone-beam computed tomography
15. Optic coherence tomography
16. Terahertz imaging
17. Multiphoton imaging
18. Infrared thermography
19. Infrared fluorescence

- **Methods of Caries Control**

The control of dental caries presents one of the greatest challenges that must be dealt with by the dental professionals.

Suggested methods of control may be classified into three general types [9]:

1. Chemical measures

   Fluoride, iodide, bis-biguanide, silver nitrate, zinc chloride and potassium ferrocyanide, vitamin K, sarcosine, urea and ammonium compounds, chlorophyll, and nitrofurans
2. Nutritional measures

   Restriction of refined carbohydrate intake and phosphated diet
3. Mechanical measures

   There are numerous means of cleansing the tooth mechanically, and these were reviewed and classified by Hine in a discussion of caries control measures as:
   - Oral prophylaxis by the dentist
   - Tooth brushing
   - Mouth rinsing
   - Use of dental floss or toothpicks
   - Incorporation of detergent foods in the diet

Conclusion

Despite the advancements in dental caries detection and prevention, it is still a common infectious disease. Even with recent dental caries research, most clinical practice is still based on treating the disease by restorative treatment once it is detected, rather than on prevention. Future education and clinical research efforts should continue to emphasize early detection and caries prevention [37].

3.2.2 *Periodontal (Gum) Disease*

Gingival and periodontal diseases, in their various forms, have afflicted humans since the dawn of history. Studies in paleopathology have indicated that destructive periodontal disease, as evidenced by bone loss, affected early humans in such diverse cultures as ancient Egypt and early pre-Columbian America. The earliest historical records dealing with medical topics reveal an awareness of periodontal disease and the need for treatment. Almost all the early writings that have been preserved have sections or chapters dealing with oral diseases, and periodontal problems comprise a significant amount of space in these writings. The relationship between calculus and periodontal disease often was considered, and underlying systemic disease was frequently postulated as a cause of periodontal disorders. However, methodic, carefully reasoned, therapeutic discussions did not exist until the Arabic surgical treatises of the Middle Ages, and modern treatment, with illustrated text and sophisticated instrumentation, did not develop until the time of Pierre Fauchard in the eighteenth century [38].

Periodontal disease is a chronic inflammatory microbial disease that ranks sixth as the most common inflammatory oral disease [39]. It affects the gingiva and can destroy the supporting tissues around the tooth such as periodontal ligament, and alveolar bone that may result in tooth loss eventually [40]. Periodontal disease is prevalent in both developed and undeveloped countries, and it affects around 90% of worldwide population. Moreover, periodontal diseases usually affect more than 50% of population over 50 years [41].

Recently, it has been proven a mutual effect of periodontal diseases and different systemic conditions. Therefore, a patient with periodontal disease can have other inflammatory conditions such as insulin resistance, coronary artery disease, and arthritis in a significant amount [42–44]. The main etiological factor for developing periodontal disease is the accumulation of the dental plaque. However, there are other risk factors for the development of periodontal disease such as genetics, smoking, age, viral infection, low immune response, pregnancy, ethnicity, and systemic diseases [45, 46].

- **Classification of Periodontal Disease**

Periodontal disease classifications are useful to help establish diagnosis, determine prognosis, and facilitate treatment planning. Different classifications of periodontal diseases have been used over the years and have been replaced as new knowledge has improved our understanding of the etiology and pathology of the diseases of the periodontium.

The classification presented here is the most accepted and was presented and discussed at the International Workshop for the Classification of the Periodontal Diseases organized by the American Academy of Periodontology in 1999 [38, 47] (Table 3.3).

Table 3.3 Classification of periodontal disease

BOX 3-1 Classification of Periodontal Diseases and Conditions

Gingival Diseases
Plaque-induced gingival diseases*
Non–plaque-induced gingival lesions

Chronic Periodontitis†
Localized
Generalized

Aggressive Periodontitis
Localized
Generalized

Periodontitis as a Manifestation of Systemic Disease

Necrotizing Periodontal Diseases
Necrotizing ulcerative gingivitis
Necrotizing ulcerative periodontitis

Abscesses of the Periodontium
Gingival abscess
Periodontal abscess
Pericoronal abscess

Periodontitis Associated With Endodontic Lesions
Endodontic–periodontal lesion
Periodontal–endodontic lesion
Combined lesion

Developmental or Acquired Deformities and Conditions
Localized tooth-related factors that predispose an individual to plaque-induced gingival diseases or periodontitis
Mucogingival deformities and conditions around the teeth
Mucogingival deformities and conditions on edentulous ridges
Occlusal trauma

*These diseases may occur on a periodontium with no attachment loss or on a periodontium with attachment loss that is stable and not progressing.

†Chronic periodontitis can be further classified on the basis of its extent and severity. As a general guide, extent can be characterized as localized (<30% of sites involved) or generalized (>30% of sites involved). Severity can be characterized on the basis of the amount of clinical attachment loss (CAL) as follows: slight, 1 or 2 mm CAL; moderate, 3 or 4 mm CAL; and severe, ≥5 mm CAL.

Data from Armitage GC: *Ann Periodontol* 4:1, 1999.

Image source [38]

- **Classification of Gingival Diseases** (Table 3.4)

- **Clinical Features of Gingivitis**

The inflammation of the gingiva results in swelling with reduction and eventual loss of normal stippling. Suppuration of the gingiva, manifested by the ability to express pus from the gingival sulcus by pressure, may occur in advanced chronic gingivitis [9, 38, 47].

- **Radiographic Features**

Chronic gingivitis, in which the inflammation is limited strictly to the gingiva, does not manifest changes in the underlying bone. When bony changes become evident, the condition is termed "periodontitis."

- **Diagnosis of Periodontal Diseases**

Although the clinical signs of gingivitis are easy to detect, it is not clear how much inflammation a person must have to be considered a gingivitis case. A universally accepted threshold for the amount or severity of gingival inflammation that must be present in an individual does not exist. In studies of gingivitis and periodontitis, a variety of indices have been used (Table 3.5).

In general, however, a gingivitis case is a person with at least mild inflammation in at least one of the gingival units that is assessed. Depending on the study, a "gingival unit" may be an anatomic structure of the gingiva, such as the interdental papilla, marginal gingiva, or attached gingiva, or it may be a gingival site defined in relation to a tooth, such as the facial, lingual, mesial, or distal gingival [9, 38].

A timely identification and diagnosis of periodontal disease is the key to the dental care. Therefore, it is always recommended that as part of routine oral examinations, dentists should also perform periodontal examination. There are several

Table 3.4 Classification of gingival diseases

BOX 3-2 Gingival Diseases

Dental-Plaque–Induced Gingival Diseases

These diseases may occur on a periodontium with no attachment loss or on a periodontium with attachment loss that is stable and not progressing.

- I. Gingivitis associated with dental plaque only
  - A. Without local contributing factors
  - B. With local contributing factors (see Box 3-4)
- II. Gingival diseases modified by systemic factors
  - A. Associated with the endocrine system
    - 1. Puberty-associated gingivitis
    - 2. Menstrual-cycle–associated gingivitis
    - 3. Pregnancy-associated conditions
      - a. Gingivitis
      - b. Pyogenic granuloma
    - 4. Diabetes-mellitus–associated gingivitis
  - B. Associated with blood dyscrasias
    - 1. Leukemia-associated gingivitis
    - 2. Other
- III. Gingival diseases modified by medications
  - A. Drug-influenced gingival diseases
    - 1. Drug-influenced gingival enlargements
    - 2. Drug-influenced gingivitis
      - a. Oral-contraceptive–associated gingivitis
      - b. Other
- IV. Gingival diseases modified by malnutrition
  - A. Ascorbic-acid–deficiency gingivitis
  - B. Other

Non–Plaque-Induced Gingival Lesions

- I. Gingival diseases of specific bacterial origin
  - A. *Neisseria gonorrhoeae*
  - B. *Treponema pallidum*
  - C. *Streptococcus* species
  - D. Other
- II. Gingival diseases of viral origin
  - A. Herpesvirus infections
    - 1. Primary herpetic gingivostomatitis
    - 2. Recurrent oral herpes
    - 3. Varicella zoster
  - B. Other
- III. Gingival diseases of fungal origin
  - A. *Candida* species infections: generalized gingival candidiasis
  - B. Linear gingival erythema
  - C. Histoplasmosis
  - D. Other
- IV. Gingival lesions of genetic origin
  - A. Hereditary gingival fibromatosis
  - B. Other
- V. Gingival manifestations of systemic conditions
  - A. Mucocutaneous lesions
    - 1. Lichen planus
    - 2. Pemphigoid
    - 3. Pemphigus vulgaris
    - 4. Erythema multiforme
    - 5. Lupus erythematosus
    - 6. Drug-induced conditions
    - 7. Other
  - B. Allergic reactions
    - 1. Dental restorative materials
      - a. Mercury
      - b. Nickel
      - c. Acrylic
      - d. Other
    - 2. Reactions attributable to the following:
      - a. Toothpastes or dentifrices
      - b. Mouth rinses or mouthwashes
      - c. Chewing-gum additives
      - d. Foods and additives
    - 3. Other
- VI. Traumatic lesions (factitious, iatrogenic, or accidental)
  - A. Chemical injury
  - B. Physical injury
  - C. Thermal injury
- VII. Foreign-body reactions
- VIII. Not otherwise specified

Data from Holmstrup P: *Ann Periodontol* 4:20, 1999; and Mariotti A: *Ann Periodontol* 4:7, 1999.

Data from Holmstrup P: *Ann Periodontol* **4:20, 1999; and Mariotti A:** *Ann Periodontol* **4:7, 1999. Image source [38]**

conventional approaches that have been used for assessment and prediction of periodontal ligament status of the individuals. For instances, periodontal risk assessment (PRA) proposed by Lange and Tonetti is one of the most widely used strategy for evaluation and predicting periodontal status of patient [48]. PRA relies on evaluating the clinical condition of the periodontal ligaments taking into consideration three important risk factors such as patient age, systemic condition, and behavioral- and environmental-related factor such as smoking [48]. However, this approach is very challenging as the dentist should have a great clinical experience. Moreover, to consider the complexity of the modifying effect of all the risk factor on the clinical status to assess and predict periodontal status of individual is an exceedingly difficult task. Artificial intelligence has been introduced for all field of dentistry and periodontal diseases were not expected. Artificial intelligence has been used for improving prediction, diagnosis, classification, and treatment of periodontal diseases. A recent study was conducted in France by Monsarrat et al., in 2022, in which

Table 3.5 Diagnostic criteria for periodontitis

Diagnostic criteria for periodontitis, according to Gomes-Filho et al.,[4] and Gomes-Filho et al., modified*

Severity Level	Probing Depth (PD)		Clinical Attachment Level	Bleeding Upon Probing
Severe Periodontitis	≥4 ≥2*	teeth with≥1 site with PD≥5mm	CAL≥5 mm on the same site	Bleeding upon stimulus
Moderate Periodontitis	≥4 ≥2*	teeth with≥1 site with PD≥4 mm	CAL≥ 3 mm on the same site	Bleeding upon stimulus
Mild Periodontitis	≥ 4 ≥2*	teeth with≥1 site with PD≥4 mm	CAL≥1 mm on the same site	Bleeding upon stimulus
No Periodontitis	Individuals who were not included in the previous groups			

*The difference between the last two criteria is only the minimum number of teeth considered: at least 2 teeth for the criterion Gomes-Filho et al.,[7] modified.

Image source [38]

the authors used machine learning algorithm combined with explainability algorithms (kernel SHAP) to predict and identify individuals with risk of developing periodontal diseases [49]. The study included five variables as the most contributive attributes used to predict periodontal health. These factors are age, systemic pathologies (mostly cardiovascular, endocrine, and metabolic diseases), hormonal status, dried vegetable or fruit consumption, and sugary drink consumption. The proposed model of prediction shows promising results of using AI-based technology in prediction and scoring the periodontal status for each individual according to their biological, clinical, and sociodemographic factors [49].

It is very acceptable that radiographs play a vital role as a tool for clinical examination in diagnosis of periodontal diseases and in planning patient's treatment [50]. The panoramic radiography has been accepted as the standard procedure for a comprehensive diagnosis and treatment planning. The benefit of panoramic radiograph is that it provides ample information to the dentist in selection of specific areas for additional intraoral periapical radiographs so that the selected tooth and the surrounding bone can be examined completely while reducing the radiation exposure to the patient [51]. The key benefit of panoramic radiographs is that they demonstrate complete dentition, which allows diagnosis of impacted teeth and detection of foreign bodies in the jaws and gross abnormalities in the number, position, and anatomy of the teeth [51]. Due to its time efficiency, patient tolerance, and low radiation exposure, the use of panoramic radiographs in the field of periodontics has been significant. In the traditional periodontal examination, periapical radiographs and periodontal probes are the regular diagnostic tools used for identifying and diagnosing periodontally compromised teeth. But this diagnostic process takes time and depends mainly on the clinical skills of the dentist [45]. Deep learning methods, as a subtype of artificial intelligence, are very advantageous in a variety of applica tions such as image processing. Deep learning has become a standard technique in medical image detection and classification with its use of convolutional neural networks (CNNs).

To use the advances of deep learning technology in periodontology, a study was conducted by Lee et al., in 2018, using a deep learning-based convolutional neural network algorithm in which 16 convolutional layers and 3 fully connected dense layers were used to predict and diagnose periodontally compromised teeth [52]. The study used periapical radiographic images of all the included patient to train the AI machine. The study showed that the deep learning algorithm has achieved 81% diagnostic accuracy for premolars and 76.7% for molars which were diagnosed as periodontally compromised teeth. In addition, the study demonstrated accuracy of predicting extraction was 82.8% for premolars and 73.4% for molars [52]. Another study was conducted by Krios et al., in 2019, who used panoramic dental radiographs as input data to train deep convolutional neural network (CNN) model to detect the amount of periodontal bone loss [53]. The final model was composed of a seven-layer deep neural network which succeeded to have accuracy rate of 81%, sensitivity rate of 81%, and specificity rate of 81% in comparison to expert dentist that showed accuracy rate of 76%, sensitivity rate of 92%, and specificity rate of 63% in detection of periodontal bone loss on the radiographs. The study concluded that using deep neural network technology showed higher discrimination ability than dentists for assessing periodontal bone loss on radiographs [53].

One of the main problems and defects related to detection of peri-implant bone loss using preapical radiograph is the difficulty to determine and identify the margins of bone around the implants. A study conducted by Jun-Young Cha et al. demonstrated the ability of using convolutional neural networks (CNNs) to assess the severity of peri-implantitis by calculating the amount of bone loss in an automatic way. In addition, the study showed the ability of CNNS to identify the anatomical landmarks around the implants such as the marginal bone level, top, and apex of implants [54]. Furthermore, another interesting study conducted by Liu et al., in 2020 in China, proposed a software based on AI technology and mobile terminal to act as chair-side and client-side connector [55]. The model was designed to be used at home by patients for enhancement and accessibility of dental treatment and prevention, early detection, and monitoring of periodontal diseases [55]. In addition, one study conducted by Huang et al., in 2020, highlighted the potentiality of using 20 periodontal disease-related proteins as a periodontal disease antibody array for easy detection and diagnosis of periodontal diseases based on machine learning classifier technology [56].

Finally, AI-based technology has been proposed to be used as a diagnostic model to help dental clinicians to take a proper decision related to treatment and prognosis of periodontal diseases. A study was conducted by Farhadian, Shokouhi, and Torkzaban in 2020 using machine learning technology in order to facilitate and accelerate diagnostic process of periodontal diseases to help less clinical experienced dentists to make an accurate precise decision [57]. The study found that using machine learning-based model, different types of periodontal conditions including gingivitis with an accurate rate of 96.0%, localized periodontitis with 64.0%, and generalized periodontitis with 92.2% were being classified [57].

- **Treatment and Prognosis**

The goal of periodontitis treatment is to thoroughly clean the pockets around teeth and prevent damage to surrounding bone. Prognosis gets better when patients adopt daily routine of good oral care, manage health conditions that may impact dental health, and stop tobacco use [58].

Nonsurgical Treatments
If periodontitis isn't advanced, treatment may involve less invasive procedures, including the following:

- **Scaling.** Scaling removes calculus and bacteria from the tooth surfaces and beneath the gingiva. It may be performed using instruments, a laser, or an ultrasonic device.
- **Root planing.** Root planing smooths the root surfaces, discouraging further buildup of plaque, calculus, and bacteria, and removes bacterial byproducts that contribute to inflammation and delay healing or reattachment of the gingiva to the tooth surfaces.
- **Antibiotics.** Topical or oral antibiotics can help control bacterial infection. Topical antibiotics can include antibiotic mouth rinses or insertion of gels containing antibiotics in the space between the teeth and gingiva or into pockets after deep cleaning. However, oral antibiotics may be necessary to completely eliminate infection-causing bacteria.

Surgical Treatments
If you have advanced periodontitis, treatment may require dental surgery, such as the following:

- **Flap surgery (pocket reduction surgery).** Tiny incisions are done on gingiva so that a section of gingival tissue can be lifted back, exposing the roots for more effective scaling and root planing. Because periodontitis often causes bone loss, the underlying bone may be recontoured before the gum tissue is sutured back in place. After you heal, it's easier to clean these areas and maintain healthy gum tissue.
- **Soft tissue grafts.** When you lose gingival tissue, your gingival recedes from its normal position. You may need to have some of the damaged soft tissue reinforced. This is usually done by removing a small amount of tissue from the roof of your mouth (palate) or using tissue from another donor source and attaching it to the affected site. This can help reduce further gingival recession, cover exposed roots, and give your teeth a more pleasing appearance.
- **Bone grafting.** This procedure is performed when periodontitis has destroyed the bone surrounding your tooth root. The graft may be composed of small fragments of your own bone, or the bone may be synthetic or donated. The bone graft

helps prevent tooth loss by holding your tooth in place. It also serves as a platform for the regrowth of natural bone.

- **Guided tissue regeneration.** This allows the regrowth of bone that was destroyed by bacteria. In one approach, your dentist places a special piece of biocompatible fabric between existing bone and your tooth. The material prevents unwanted tissue from entering the healing area, allowing bone to grow back instead.
- **Tissue-stimulating proteins.** Another technique involves applying a special gel to a diseased tooth root. This gel contains the same proteins found in developing tooth enamel and stimulates the growth of healthy bone and tissue [58].

3.2.3 Oral Cancer

The study of tumors of the oral cavity and adjacent structures constitutes an important phase of dentistry because of the role which the dentist plays in the diagnosis and treatment of these lesions. Although tumors constitute only a small number of the pathologic conditions seen by the dentist, they are of great significance since they have the potential ability to jeopardize the health and longevity of the patient.

A tumor, by definition, is simply a swelling of the tissue in the strict sense; the word does not imply a neoplastic process. A neoplasm can be defined as an abnormal mass of tissue, the growth of which exceeds and is uncoordinated with that of the normal tissues and persists in the same excessive manner after cessation of the stimuli which evoked the change [9].

Oral cancers are most often discovered after they have spread to the lymph nodes of neck. Early detection is key to surviving oral cancer.

Oral cancers include cancers of the [59]:

- Lips
- Tongue
- Inner lining of the cheek
- Gums
- Floor of the mouth
- Hard and soft palate

Risk Factors for Developing Oral Cancer

One of the biggest risk factors for oral cancer is tobacco use. This includes smoking cigarettes, cigars, and pipes, as well as chewing tobacco. People who consume large amounts of alcohol and tobacco are at an even greater risk, especially when both products are used on a regular basis [9].

Other risk factors include:

- Human papillomavirus (HPV) infection
- Chronic facial sun exposure
- A previous diagnosis of oral cancer
- A family history of oral or other types of cancer

- A weakened immune system
- Poor nutrition
- Genetic syndromes
- Being male

Men are twice as likely to get oral cancer compared to women [60].
Symptoms of oral cancer include:

- A sore on your lip or mouth that won't heal
- A mass or growth anywhere in your mouth
- Bleeding from your mouth
- Loose teeth
- Pain or difficulty swallowing
- Trouble wearing dentures
- A lump in your neck
- An earache that won't go away
- Dramatic weight loss
- Lower lip, face, neck, or chin numbness
- White, red and white, or red patches in or on your mouth or lips
- A sore throat
- Jaw pain or stiffness
- Tongue pain

Some of these symptoms, such as a sore throat or an earache, may indicate other conditions. However, if it persists, it needs immediate attention [61].

- **Diagnosis of Oral Cancer**

There are many tests used for diagnosing oral or oropharyngeal cancer. Not all tests described here will be used for every person. The doctor may consider these factors when choosing a diagnostic test [61, 62]:

- The type of cancer suspected
- Patient's signs and symptoms
- Patient's age and general health
- The results of earlier medical tests

The following tests may be used to diagnose oral or oropharyngeal cancer:

- **Physical examination.** Dentists and doctors often find lip and oral cavity cancers during routine checkups. If a person shows signs of oral or oropharyngeal cancer, the doctor will take a complete medical history, asking about the patient's symptoms and risk factors. The doctor will feel for any lumps on the neck, lips, gums, and cheeks. Because people with oral or oropharyngeal cancer have a higher risk of other cancers elsewhere in the head and neck region, the doctor will examine the area behind the nose, the larynx (voice box), and the lymph nodes of the neck.
- **Endoscopy.** An endoscopy allows the doctor to see inside the mouth and throat. Typically, a thin, flexible tube with an attached light and view lens, called an

endoscope, is inserted through the nose to examine the head and neck areas. Sometimes, a rigid endoscope, which is a hollow tube with a light and view lens, is placed into the back of the mouth to see the back of the throat in more detail.

- Endoscopic examinations have different names depending on the area of the body that is examined, such as laryngoscopy to view the larynx, pharyngoscopy to view the pharynx, or nasopharyngoscopy to view the nasopharynx. To make the patient more comfortable, these examinations are performed using an anesthetic spray to numb the area. If an area looks suspicious, the doctor will take a biopsy. Tests are often done in the doctor's office. However, sometimes an endoscopy must be performed in an operating room at a hospital using general anesthesia, which blocks the awareness of pain.
- **Biopsy.** A biopsy is the removal of a small amount of tissue for examination under a microscope. Other tests can suggest that cancer is present, but only a biopsy can make a definite diagnosis. The type of biopsy performed will depend on the location of the cancer. During a fine needle aspiration biopsy, cells are removed using a thin needle inserted directly into the suspicious area. A pathologist then analyzes the cells. A pathologist is a doctor who specializes in interpreting laboratory tests and evaluating cells, tissues, and organs to diagnose disease.
- **Oral brush biopsy**. During routine dental examinations, some dentists are using a newer, simple technique to detect oral cancer in which the dentist uses a small brush to gather cell samples of a suspicious area. The specimen is then sent to a laboratory for analysis. This procedure can be done in the dentist's chair with very little or no pain. If cancer is found using this method, a traditional biopsy is recommended to confirm the results.
- **HPV testing.** HPV testing may be done on a sample of the tumor removed during the biopsy. As described in Risk Factors and Prevention, HPV has been linked to a higher risk of oropharyngeal cancer. Knowing if a person has HPV can help determine the cancer's stage and the treatment options that are likely to be most effective.
- **X-ray.** An x-ray is a way to picturize the structures inside of the body, using a small amount of radiation. X-rays may be recommended by the dentist or doctor to look for abnormal findings in the mouth or neck.
- **Barium swallow/modified barium swallow**. There are two barium swallow tests that are generally used to look at the oropharynx and to check a patient's swallowing. The first is a traditional barium swallow. During an x-ray exam, the patient is asked to swallow liquid barium. This lets the doctor look for any changes in the structure of the oral cavity and throat and see whether the liquid passes easily to the stomach. A modified barium swallow, or video fluoroscopy, may be used to evaluate difficulties with swallowing.
- **Computed tomography (CT or CAT) scan.** A CT scan takes pictures of the inside of the body using x-rays taken from different angles. A computer combines these pictures into a detailed, three-dimensional image that shows any abnormalities or tumors. A CT scan can be used to measure the tumor's size, help the doctor decide whether the tumor can be surgically removed, and show whether the cancer has spread to lymph nodes in the neck or lower jawbone.

Sometimes, a special dye called a contrast medium is given before the scan to provide better detail on the image. This dye can be injected into a patient's vein or given as a pill or liquid to swallow.

- **Magnetic resonance imaging (MRI).** An MRI uses magnetic fields, not x-rays, to produce detailed images of the body, especially images of soft tissue, such as the tonsils and the base of the tongue. MRI can be used to measure the tumor's size. A special dye called a contrast medium is given before the scan to create a clearer picture. This dye can be injected into a patient's vein or given as a pill or liquid to swallow.
- **Ultrasound.** An ultrasound uses sound waves to create a picture of the internal organs. This test can detect the spread of cancer to the lymph nodes in the neck, which doctors also call the "cervical lymph nodes."
- **Positron emission tomography (PET) or PET-CT scan.** A PET scan is usually combined with a CT scan, called a PET-CT scan. However, you may hear your doctor refer to this procedure just as a PET scan. A PET scan is a way to create pictures of organs and tissues inside the body. A small amount of a radioactive sugar substance is injected into the patient's body. This sugar substance is taken up by cells that use the most energy. Because cancer tends to use energy actively, it absorbs more of the radioactive substance. However, the amount of radiation in the substance is too low to be harmful. A scanner then detects this substance to produce images of the inside of the body [62].

It is well known that oral cancer has the worst prognosis and survival rate among all type of cancers. According to the report of the American Academy of Oral Medicine published in 2019, there is approximately 52,000 individuals diagnosed as new cases with oral cancers, among them around 11,000 related deaths annually. The facts that placed oral cancer to rank the sixth position as the most common type of cancers in the United States [63]. Oropharyngeal squamous cell carcinoma (OPSCC), a type of oral cancer, is the most frequent type of oral cancer comprising 90% of the condition [64]. According to the recent studies, there are almost 640,000 new cases annually diagnosed of OPSCC worldwide. Most of these cases (approximately two-thirds) localized in the countries with low and middle incomes [65].

Early diagnosed OPSCC has almost 80% 5-year survival rate for US patients; however, late diagnosed cases with metastasis have only 20–30% survival rate [66]. Therefore, early diagnosis and identification of the disease are very critical for the improvement prognosis of the diseases. Globally, different governments are trying to conduct several community and company activities to increase awareness and knowledge of the risk factors and symptoms of the disease to enhance early diagnosis of the conditions [67]. Nowadays, it has been proved that tobacco and alcohol consumptions are the primary causes of OPSCC [68]. However, in certain countries such as Europe and North America, there is a wide spread of human papillomavirus (HPV) infection that can be associated with oral cancer adding more burden for such countries [69]. Unfortunately, most of the cases of oral cancers are asymptomatic in the early stages (Stage I and Stage II) and easy to be missed and detected at late stages (Stage II and Stage III). It has been reported that more than 60% of all oral cancers are detected in the late stages that have a very bad outcomes including high morbidity and mortality [65].

According to the National Center for Health Statistics, over than 60% of adults visit a dentist each year [70]. This fact has made dentists as the first health-care profession to detect the oral cancers during providing routine dental care [63]. Indeed, the American Academy of Oral Medicine is recommending a comprehensive assessment of the risk factors of oral cancer with a proper visual and tactile examination of oral mucosa during routine dental visit by any dental specialist [63]. This routine behavior can increase early detection of oral cancers and leads to a referral of positive cases for more confirmatory tests such as histological biopsy. By this way, dentists can be playing an effective role as a gatekeeper for detection and diagnosis of oral cancers. However, there are several factors that act as barriers to enable dentist to play such a crucial role including insufficient knowledge and practice of dentists to recognize and diagnose premalignant and malignant oral lesions.

Moreover, most of dentists are relying on subjective examinations and analyses of clinical findings such as consistency, shape, color, and texture of the lesion [71]. Another important issue that affects the ability of dentists to diagnose and detect oral cancers early is their low competent level in taking biopsy which is mandatory for final confirmation of oral cancers [72]. These main factors lead to poor and inaccurate screening by dentists [71].

Artificial intelligence-based technology can provide a tool for collecting and analyzing very complex and diverse amount of data including clinical findings in a standardized way. These subjective immense information and reports can help dentists for improving their decisions minimizing the variations due to knowledge or clinical experience that will have great impact on outcomes of the disease [73]. For example, AI-based machines can assist dentists to monitor longitudinally any change in the oral premalignant liaisons (OPMLs) in a manner that can raise an alert whether a referral to another specialist may be required. Furthermore, imaging processing and analysis for many biomarkers related to formation, metastases, or regression of tumors such as blood flow, level of oxygenation, metabolic rates, cell viability, and tissue architecture can provide easy screening and early detection of such neoplasms [74].

Conventional imaging approaches for screening oral tissues have been used for easy and early detection of oral cancers. For example, autofluorescence imaging has been validated by several studies to be used as an adjunctive method for detection and distinguishing between oral cancer and premalignant lesions [75]. Recently, advances of AI-based imaging technology improved the drawbacks and pitfalls of conventional imaging. Optical coherence tomography (OCT) was introduced as an AI-based imaging technique in 1991. OCT technology is using the reflected light as backscattered signals reflected from the tissue to reconstruct structural images. OCT can generate three-dimensional images that can be used for reconstruction of the target tissue and proper examination and diagnosis of the tumor.

More recently, AI-based imaging techniques have been improved giving better results in screening oral cancers. For example, a clinical study using deep learning-supported smartphone to screen oral cancers in 92 subjects with oral lesions gave an accuracy rate of 80.6% when it is compared with standard-of-care diagnosis [76]. The success of improving the accuracy of deep learning-based technology for detection of oral cancer has encouraged more studies to investigate the OCT technology in detection and diagnosis of oral cancers, for example, providing OCT imaging system with a diagnostic algorithm led to easy interpretation of the OCT images. Using the advantage of this technology, a recent study used an automated cancer screening platform to differentiate between normal, malignant, and dysplastic lesions. The study showed sensitivity of 87% and a specificity of 83% versus the histopathological gold standard [77].

- **Treatment of Oral Cancer**

Oral and oropharyngeal cancers can often be cured, especially if the cancer is found at an early stage. Although curing the cancer is the primary goal of treatment, preserving the function of the nearby nerves, organs, and tissues is also very important. When doctors plan treatment, they consider how treatment might affect a person's quality of life, such as how the person feels, looks, talks, eats, and breathes [61, 62].

In many cases, a team of doctors will work together with the patient to create the best treatment plan. Head and neck cancer specialists often form a multidisciplinary team to care for each patient. This team may include the following:

- **Medical oncologist:** A doctor who treats cancer using chemotherapy or other medications, such as targeted therapy and immunotherapy.
- **Radiation oncologist:** A doctor who specializes in treating cancer using radiation therapy.
- **Surgical oncologist:** A doctor who treats cancer using surgery.
- **Otolaryngologist:** A doctor who specializes in the ear, nose, and throat.
- **Reconstructive/plastic surgeon:** A doctor who specializes in reconstructive surgery, which is done to help repair damage caused by cancer treatment.
- **Maxillofacial prosthodontist:** A specialist who performs restorative surgery in the head and neck areas.
- **Oncologic dentist or oral oncologist:** Dentists experienced in caring for people with head and neck cancer.
- **Prosthodontist:** A dental specialist with expertise in the restoration and replacement of broken teeth with crowns, bridges, or dentures.
- **Physical therapist:** A health-care professional who helps patients improve their physical strength and ability to move.
- **Speech-language pathologist:** A health-care professional who specializes in communication and swallowing disorders. A speech-language pathologist helps patients regain their speaking, swallowing, and oral motor skills after cancer treatment that affects the head, mouth, and neck.
- **Audiologist:** A health-care professional who treats and manages hearing problems that may be caused by the tumor itself or the cancer treatment.

- **Psychologist/psychiatrist:** These mental health professionals address the emotional, psychological, and behavioral needs of the person with cancer and those of their family.

Cancer care teams include a variety of other health-care professionals, such as physician assistants, nurse practitioners, oncology nurses, social workers, pharmacists, counselors, dietitians, and others. It is extremely important for the team to create a comprehensive treatment plan before treatment begins. People may need to be seen by several specialists before a treatment plan is fully developed.

There are three main treatment options for oral and oropharyngeal cancer: surgery, radiation therapy, and therapies using medication.

Treatment options and recommendations depend on several factors, including the type and stage of cancer, possible side effects, and the patient's preferences and overall health. One of these therapies, or a combination of them, may be used.

Surgery Surgery is the removal of the tumor and some surrounding healthy tissue, known as a margin, during an operation. An important goal of the surgery is the complete removal of the tumor with "negative margins." Negative margins means that there is no trace of cancer in the margin's healthy tissue. Surgeons are often able to tell in the operating room if all of the tumor has been removed.

Sometimes surgery is followed by radiation therapy, therapies using medication, or both. Depending on the location, stage, grade, and other features of the cancer, some people may need more than one operation to remove the cancer and to help restore the appearance and function of the affected tissues.

The most common surgical procedures for the removal of oral or oropharyngeal cancer include the following:

- **Primary tumor surgery.** The tumor and a margin of healthy tissue around it are removed to decrease the chance that any cancerous cells will be left behind. The tumor may be removed through the mouth or through an incision in the neck. A mandibulotomy, in which the jawbone is split to allow the surgeon to reach the tumor, may also be required.
- **Glossectomy.** This is the partial or total removal of the tongue.
- **Mandibulectomy.** If the tumor has entered a jawbone but not spread into the bone, then a piece of the jawbone or the whole jawbone will be removed. If there is evidence of destruction of the jawbone on an x-ray, then the entire bone may need to be removed.
- **Maxillectomy.** This surgery removes part or all of the hard palate, which is the bony roof of the mouth. Prosthesis (an artificial replacement), or more recently, the use of flaps of soft tissue with and without bone, can be placed to fill gaps created during this operation.
- **Neck dissection.** Cancer of the oral cavity or oropharynx often spreads to lymph nodes in the neck. Preventing the cancer from spreading to the lymph nodes is an important goal of treatment. It may be necessary to remove some or all of these lymph nodes using a surgical procedure called a neck dissection, even if the lymph nodes show no evidence of cancer when examined. A neck dissection may

be followed by radiation therapy or a combination of chemotherapy and radiation therapy, called chemoradiation, to make sure there is no cancer remaining in the lymph nodes. Sometimes, for oropharyngeal cancer, a neck dissection will be recommended after radiation therapy or chemoradiation. If a neck dissection is not possible, radiation therapy may be used instead.

- **Laryngectomy.** A laryngectomy is the complete or partial removal of the larynx or voice box. Although the larynx is important for producing sounds, the larynx is also critical to swallowing because it protects the airway from food and liquid entering the trachea or windpipe and reaching the lungs, which can cause pneumonia. A laryngectomy is rarely needed to treat oral or oropharyngeal cancer. However, when there is a large tumor of the tongue or oropharynx, the doctor may need to remove the larynx to protect the airway during swallowing. If the larynx is removed, the windpipe is reattached to the skin of the neck where a hole, called a stoma or tracheostomy, is made. Rehabilitation will be needed to learn a new way of speaking.
- **Transoral robotic surgery and transoral laser microsurgery.** Transoral robotic surgery (TORS) and transoral laser microsurgery (TLM) are minimally invasive surgical procedures. This means that they do not require large cuts to get to and remove a tumor. In TORS, an endoscope is used to see a tumor in the throat, the base of the tongue, and the tonsils. Then two small robotic instruments act as the surgeon's arms to remove the tumor. In TLM, an endoscope connected to a laser is inserted through the mouth. The laser is then used to remove the tumor. A laser is a narrow beam of high-intensity light.
- Other types of surgery may also be needed, including the following:
  - **Micrographic surgery.** This type of surgery is frequently used to treat skin cancer and can sometimes be used for oral cavity tumors. It can reduce the amount of healthy tissue removed. This technique is often used with cancer of the lip. It involves removing the visible tumor in addition to small fragments of tissue surrounding the tumor. Each small fragment is examined under a microscope until all of the cancer has been removed.
  - **Tracheostomy.** If cancer is blocking the airway or is too large to completely remove, a hole is made in the neck. This hole is called a tracheostomy. A tracheostomy tube is then placed, and a person breathes through this tube. A tracheostomy can be temporary or permanent.
  - **Gastrostomy tube.** If cancer prevents a person from swallowing, a feeding device called a gastrostomy tube is placed. The tube goes through the skin and muscle of the abdomen and directly into the stomach. These tubes may be used as a temporary method for maintaining nutrition until the person can safely and adequately swallow food taken in through the mouth. For swallowing problems that are temporary, a nasogastric (NG) tube may be used instead of a tube into the stomach. An NG tube is inserted through the nose, down the esophagus, and into the stomach.
  - **Reconstruction.** If treatment requires removing large areas of tissue, reconstructive surgery may be necessary to help the patient swallow and speak

Nutrition is also an important part of oral cancer treatment. Many treatments make it difficult or painful to eat and swallow, and poor appetite and weight loss are common.

Getting the advice of a nutritionist can help in planning a food menu that will be gentle on the mouth and throat, and will provide the body with calories, vitamins, and minerals it needs to heal [38].

Finally, **keeping the mouth healthy** and moist during cancer treatments is a crucial part of treatment.

- **Recovering from Oral Cancer Treatment**

The recovery from each type of treatment will vary. Post-surgery symptoms can include pain and swelling, but removing small tumors usually has no associated long-term problems.

The removal of larger tumors could possibly affect the ability to chew, swallow, or talk as it was done before the surgery. Patient might also need reconstructive surgery to rebuild the bones and tissues in their face removed during surgery.

Radiation therapy can have a negative effect on the body. Some of the side effects of radiation include:

- A sore throat or mouth
- Dry mouth and loss of salivary gland function
- Tooth decay
- Nausea and vomiting
- Sore or bleeding gums
- Skin and mouth infections
- Jaw stiffness and pain
- Problems wearing dentures
- Fatigue
- A change in your ability to taste and smell
- Changes in your skin, including dryness and burning
- Weight loss
- Thyroid changes

Chemotherapy drugs can be toxic to rapidly growing noncancerous cells. This can cause side effects such as:

- Hair loss
- Painful mouth and gums
- Bleeding in the mouth
- Severe anemia
- Weakness
- Poor appetite
- Nausea
- Vomiting
- Diarrhea
- Mouth and lip sores

- Numbness in the hands and feet

Recovering from targeted therapies is usually minimal. The side effects of this treatment can include:

- Fever
- Headache
- Vomiting
- Diarrhea
- An allergic reaction
- Skin rashes

Although these treatments do have side effects, they're often necessary in beating the cancer.

Reconstruction and Rehabilitation After Oral Cancer Treatment
People who are diagnosed with advanced oral cancer will likely need reconstructive surgery and some rehabilitation to assist with eating and speaking during recovery.

Reconstruction can involve dental implants or grafts to repair the missing bones and tissues in the mouth or face. Artificial palates are used to replace any missing tissue or teeth.

Rehabilitation is also necessary for cases of advanced cancer. Speech therapy can be provided from the time the patients get out of surgery until they reach the maximum level of improvement.

The outlook for oral cancers depends on the specific type and stage of cancer at diagnosis. It also depends on your general health, your age, and your tolerance and response to treatment. Early diagnosis is critical because treating Stage I and Stage II cancers may be less involved and have a higher chance of successful treatment [61, 62].

3.2.4 Oral Manifestation of HIV Infection

Acquired immunodeficiency syndrome (AIDS) is caused by the human immunodeficiency virus (HIV) and is characterized by immunosuppression, which leads to a spectrum of clinical manifestations that include opportunistic infections, secondary neoplasms, and neurologic manifestations. Two genetically distinct populations of viruses known to cause AIDS are HIV-1 and HIV-2. HIV-1 is the most common type responsible for AIDS in Central Africa and the rest of the world, and HIV-2 in West Africa and India [9].

- **Epidemiology**

HIV infection was first reported in the mid-1981 in New York City, when young homosexual men showed Kaposi's sarcoma and unusual clusters of pneumocystis carinii pneumonia [78]. Since this time, HIV/AIDS infection became one of the major causes of death worldwide. Currently, human immunodeficiency virus (HIV)/

acquired immunodeficiency syndrome (AIDS) is ranked as the fourth leading cause of death worldwide [79]. In the United States, it was estimated that almost 40,000 people get infected with HIV each year, while globally in 2018, it was estimated that around 1.7 million new cases were reported [80].

Estimates at the end of 2007 indicate that there are 33 million people living with HIV infection, 2.7 million have new infection, and 2.0 million have succumbed to the disease. Ninety-six percent of the infected are in low- and middle-income countries. The demographic features of the spread of HIV in Asia are somewhat different from that in other parts of the world, as the infection was first seen in intravenous drug users (IDUs) in Thailand and Burma in contrast to groups indulging in high-risk sexual behavior in the western countries. Globally, South and Southeast Asian countries follow South Africa in terms of the total number of people living with the disease (UNAIDS).

The UAE ranks as number one in the world for the lowest prevalence of HIV (per percentage of the adult population). The first cases of HIV in the UAE emerged in reports in the 1980s and reached a cumulative total of 780 cases among UAE national citizens by the end of 2012. According to the World Health Organization, the number of new HIV cases per year increased from 25 in 2010 to 49 in 2016, which, despite the increase, remains significantly low [81].

- **Mode of HIV Transmission**

Sexual transmission is the predominant mode of infection worldwide, accounting for more than 75% of all cases of HIV transmission. It is also transmitted through infected body fluids such as blood and blood products, and breast milk. HIV has been demonstrated in oral fluids, but their infectivity appears to be reduced. So, saliva is not a significant route of transmission of HIV infection. Infection can be transmitted vertically from mother to the child [9].

- **Pathogenesis of HIV Infection**

The two major targets of HIV infections are the immune system and the central nervous system. A characteristic feature of AIDS is the profound immunosuppression of cell-mediated immunity. After gaining entry into the host, either through exposure to blood, body fluids, or sexual activity, the first step in virus infection involves binding of the virion to the surface of a target cell. This is mediated by binding of the envelope gp120 to the CD4 surface protein found on most helper T cells. After binding, the virus becomes internalized into the host cell where it becomes uncoated. The viral RNA is then reverse transcribed into linear double-stranded viral DNA in the cytoplasm of infected cells by the reverse transcriptase and then transported to the nucleus, where it is first "circularized" and then integrated into the host cell. The integrated viral DNA is transcribed into full-length RNA by the host cell. These RNA transcripts can either be packaged within virus particles, to serve as the genome of progeny virus, or they can serve as mRNA for the synthesis of viral gene products.

The most common signs and symptoms of acute infection include fever, fatigue, maculopapular rash, headache, lymphadenopathy, pharyngitis, myalgia, arthralgia, aseptic meningitis, retroorbital pain, weight loss, depression, gastrointestinal distress, night sweats, and oral or genital ulcers. The acute illness may last from a few days to more than 10 weeks, but the duration is usually less than 13 days.

The severity and the duration of the illness may have prognostic implication; severe and prolonged symptoms are correlated with rapid disease progression [9].

- **Clinical Features**

The clinical features of HIV infection range from asymptomatic infection to severe clinical illness and AIDS. The time for the onset of symptoms varies from 5 to 6 months to few years and may be influenced by the source of HIV infection, patient's age, gender, drug habits, immunogenetics, and other factors. In 1993, the Centers for Disease Control and Prevention (CDC) revised their classification system proposed in 1986 and expanded the surveillance case definition for AIDS among adolescents and adult.

Patients generally remain asymptomatic until their CD4 cell count falls below 500 cells/mm^3, at which time the patient enters the "symptomatic HIV infection" previously known as the "AIDS-related complex" and more recently referred to as "Stage B," according to the 1993 CDC classification, which is characterized by the development of opportunistic infections. As HIV continues to replicate, the CD4 cell count dramatically decreases. AIDS is diagnosed when the CD4 cell count falls below 200 cells/mm^3 or when one of the AIDS defining illnesses is documented. Eventually, the immune function ceases, resulting in advanced HIV infection, characterized by a CD4 cell count <50 cells/mm^3, overwhelming opportunistic infections, and death. Without antiretroviral therapy, the progression of HIV from transmission to death is approximately 10–12 years [9] (Table 3.6).

- **Oral Lesions in HIV Infection**

Several oral lesions are considered cardinal signs for HIV/AIDS infection and usually are associated with the disease progression. These oral lesions include hairy leukoplakia, linear gingival erythema, oral candidiasis, necrotizing ulcerative periodontitis, necrotizing ulcerative gingivitis, non-Hodgkin's lymphoma (NHL), aphthous ulcer, oral submucous fibrosis, herpes zoster, exfoliative cheilitis, xerostomia,

Table 3.6 1993 revised classification system for HIV infection and expanded AIDS surveillance case definition for adolescents and adults

CD4+ T Cell Categories	Clinical Categories		
	A Asymptomatic, Acute (primary) HIV or PGL	B Symptomatic, Not A or C Condition	C AIDS-Indicator Conditions
1. ≥500/μl	A1	B1	C1
2. 200 ~ 499/μl	A2	B2	C2
3.<200/μl	A3	B3	C3

Image source [38]

and salivary gland disease [82]. The prevalence of oral lesions in HIV-infected patients has been reported in 70–90% of HIV-positive patients [83].

Oral lesions are often clearly visible and several can be diagnosed accurately on clinical features alone. In those cases where HIV status is unknown and where HIV testing is difficult, certain oral lesions provide a strong indication of the presence of HIV infection. Oral lesions that are associated with this disease are important, as they not only affect the quality of life of the patient but also are useful markers of disease progression and immunosuppression. They are strongly associated with immunosuppression, as measured by CD4 cell counts, and are modestly associated with a high viral burden. Thus, oropharyngeal lesions feature in all classifications, staging, and prognosis. Oral lesions have also been advocated and are used as entry criteria and end points for prophylaxis therapy and vaccine trials [9] (Table 3.7).

In 1995, European Commission (EC) Clearinghouse on oral problems related to HIV infection and the WHO Collaborating Center on oral manifestations of the immunodeficiency virus released the following classification:

- Presumptive criteria: Relate to the initial clinical appearance of the lesion.
- Definitive criteria: They are the result of special investigations for absolute diagnosis.

These two added criteria give the diagnostic criteria of the oral manifestations of HIV infection [9].

- **Diagnosis of HIV**

Detection and diagnosis of the HIV infection are very critical to prevent transmission of the diseases. Counting the CD4+ lymphocyte is the gold standard laboratory marker used for detection of and monitoring HIV disease and progression. However, oral clinical manifestations of HIV/AIDS can be an important and early indicator to diagnosis of HIV infection in case the CD4+ test is not available or patient is asymptomatic. The accessibility of the oral cavity has made oral clinical manifestation of AIDS/HIV playing an important role in early diagnosis, detection, and even prediction of the prognosis of the HIV infection among children and adults [82].

Advances of AI-based technology have improved clinical care of most of the infectious diseases including HIV infection. Without the improvement in prediction, diagnosis, classification, and appropriate treatment plan achieved by such technology, the humanity could not achieve such progress in health care of infectious diseases. Three studies have used AI-based technology such as machine learning and prediction algorithm to predict individuals who are at high risks for HIV infection [84]. A study conducted by Krakower et al., in 2019, has used more than 180 different patient electronic health-care records as variables to train machine learning algorithm to predict patients who are at high risks of HIV infection to support and provide them with specific HIV pre-exposure prophylaxis (PrEP) programs [85]. The second study conducted by Marcus et al. has used 81 different patient electronic health-care records for 3.7 million uninfected patients, in North Carolina, as variables to feed absolute shrinkage and selection operator (LASSO) regression model

Table 3.7 Revised classification of HIV infection (1993)

Group 1:	**Lesions strongly associated with HIV infection**
	Candidiasis
	Erythematous
	Pseudomembranous
	Hairy leukoplakia
	Kaposi's sarcoma
	Non-Hodgkin's lymphoma
	Periodontal disease
	Linear gingival erythema
	Necrotizing ulcerative gingivitis
	Necrotizing ulcerative periodontitis
Group 2:	**Lesions less commonly associated with HIV infection**
	Bacterial infections
	Mycobacterium avium–intercellulare
	Mycobacterium tuberculosis
	Melanotic hyperpigmentation
	Necrotizing ulcerative stomatitis
Group 3:	**Lesions seen in HIV infection**
	Bacterial infections
	Actinomyces israelii
	Escherichia coli
	Klebsiella pneumoniae
	Cat-scratch disease
	Drug reactions (ulcerative, erythema multiforme,
	Lichenoid reaction, toxic epidermolysis)
	Epithelioid (bacillary) angiomatosis
	Fungal infections other than candidiasis
	Cryptococcus neoformans
	Geotrichum candidum
	Histoplasma capsulatum
	Mucormycosis (zygomycosis)
	Aspergillus flavus
	Neurologic disturbances
	Facial palsy
	Trigeminal neuralgia
	Recurrent aphthous stomatitis (RAS)
	Viral infections
	CMV
	Molluscum contagiosum

Image source [38]

[86]. The author found that predictor algorithm model retained 44 variables of HER including male sex, local area, urine methadone test, and number of positive tests as a validated predictive variable to detect patient who are at high risk for HIV infection with AUC of 84%. To compare the importance of including the 44 variables, the same author compares the final algorithm model predictive performance using only variables related to sexual orientation and sexually transmitted infections (STIs). The author found that the model has higher AUC and sensitivity but lower positive predictive value [86]. The third study conducted by Ahlström et al. (2019) has used nationwide electronic registry data of 4,384,178 individuals to train machine learning algorithm to predict individuals who are at high risk of HIV infection trying to enhance early diagnosis of the disease [84]. The study suggested that the proposed predictive machine learning algorithms can learn from electronic registry data and help to predict HIV status with a fairly high level of accuracy [86].

Combining AI-based technology to smartphones and social media has offered great opportunity to monitor patient and enhance patient-doctor contact in real time for immediate advice [87]. A study was conducted by Wray et al. in 2019 who collected and assessed in a real-time manner the sexual activity of individuals on daily bases and predict unsafe sexual behavior by using machine learning. The study suggested that by this way, a reduction of 74% of unsafe sexual practice can be achieved through real-time text messages through smartphone which reduce HIV risks. Another study conducted by Young, Yu, and Wang in 2017 used social media as Twitter to collect data in a real time to feed and train machine learning applications to predict individuals who are at high risk of HIV infection [88].

There are several studies proposing other applications of AI-based technology to enhance preventive measures of HIV infection. Virtual reality and chatbots are the main tools that are proposed by these studies [89]. For example, one study was conducted by Muessig et al., using Tough Talks virtual reality program in which a focus group with HIV disease were interviewed about their sero-disclosure experiences. The author suggested that virtual reality program based on AI technology can increase and enhance protective behaviors of young MSM against HIV transmission through role-play HIV serostatus disclosure. Chatbots are another application where specific agents through which individuals can engage anonymously using different types of conversations such as messaging (text, voice). Chatbots are using AI-based application not only to maintain and collect information related to HIV diseases but also to help people who are at high risk for HIV infection to take the right decision to get the benefit form PrEP program and antiretroviral therapy [89].

Oral Lesions and Highly Active Antiretroviral Therapy (HAART)
With the introduction of HAART, there has been a decrease in the opportunistic infections associated with HIV infection [9].

Studies examining the effect of HAART on the prevalence of individual oral manifestations mainly reported on oral candidiasis, oral hairy leukoplakia, HIV-related periodontal diseases, Kaposi's sarcoma (KS), oral papilloma, and HIV-related salivary gland disease showed reduction in the prevalence [90].

Oral candidiasis (OC) has been shown to be one of the most common oral lesions in HIV patients. With the advent of HAART, most studies reported a decrease in the prevalence of oral candidiasis.

The prevalence of HIV-associated periodontal diseases was reported to decrease significantly in an American cohort, from 4.8% to 1.7% with HAART, in concordance with findings in other studies.

Kaposi's sarcoma (KS) is one of the oral manifestations that is strongly associated with HIV, although its prevalence is quite low in this groupCeballos-Salobrena et al. [9]. Studies from the United States Patton et al. [9] and Mexico (Ramírez-Amador et al. [9] found no significant change in the occurrence of Kaposi's sarcoma with HAART.

Unlike most other oral manifestations of HIV, studies from the United States and the United Kingdom (UK) described an increase in the prevalence of oral warts with HAART Patton et al. [9]; Greenwood et al. [9], which may reach statistical significance Greenspan et al. [9]. Others looking at a different population (Mexicans) reported similar detection rates of oral warts, papillomas, condylomas, and focal epithelial hyperplasia in HIV-positive subjects on HAART compared with those not on therapy (Ramírez-Amador et al. [9]).

Other lesions that are showing a trend of rising prevalence include HIV-related salivary gland disease (Patton et al. [9]). However, this was not supported by other studies (Ramírez-Amador et al. [9]). Studies from industrialized world report a decreased frequency of HIV-related oral manifestations of 10–50% following the introduction of HAART [9, 90].

3.2.5 *Oro-dental Trauma*

Oro-dental trauma results from injury to the teeth, mouth, and oral cavity. Treatment is costly and lengthy and sometimes can even lead to tooth loss, resulting in complications for facial and psychological development and quality of life [4].

Oro-dental trauma/traumatic dental injury is a very common condition in both children and adult that can take place due to several reasons such as fall, sports injury, or accident. However, traumatic dental injuries (TDIs) can take place due to certain bad habits such as chewing very hard objects such as ice cubes, holding pen, paper clips, or opening bottles cans by the teeth. TDIs are one of the most common reasons in children to visit pediatric clinics seeking dental treatment, and the oral injuries were reported to be the second most common area of injuries in the age of 1–4 years with prevalence rate ranging up to 33% [91]. It is estimated that 40% of children visit dentists for the first time due to TDIs [92]. In addition, oral traumatic injuries are considered the fourth most common type of injuries among adults from 15 to 35 that usually lead to jaw facture.

Dental trauma is physical injury to the teeth, gums, the alveolar bone (the bone that holds the tooth sockets), or the soft tissue of the mouth, including the lips and tongue. There are several types of injury that fall under the category of dental trauma, including the following [93]:

- Chipped tooth
- Tooth fractures, including root fractures, enamel fractures, etc.
- Tooth knocked loose (subluxation)
- Tooth jammed into socket (intrusion)
- Tooth knocked out (avulsion)
- Fracture of the tooth socket wall
- Jaw fracture
- Lacerations of the lips
- Lacerations of the gums

Dental trauma (traumatic dental injury) is usually sudden, circumstantial, unexpected, and accidental and often requires emergency attention. It is not a disease but a consequence of several unavoidable risk factors in life. Although these injuries are more common in certain groups, no individual is ever at zero risk through their activities of daily living [94].

Dental trauma is often more time consuming and costly compared with many other accidental injuries presenting to emergency clinics and hospitals. Trauma to the body, inclusive of the oral cavity, is a significant public health problem worldwide. In certain groups, dental trauma is almost as high as one-fifth of all bodily injuries.

Bodily injuries have been reported to be the leading cause of death among young people aged between 12 and 24 years of age. In some western countries, the direct (treatment) and indirect (lost productivity and wages, transport cost, and quality of life) cost of trauma has been estimated to be around 4–5% of gross domestic product.

In the United States alone, the lifetime cost of bodily injuries has been estimated to be US$406 billion. It has been reported that traumatic dental injuries and their consequences may exceed the burden of caries and periodontal disease in the young population [94].

- **Etiology**

Despite local and methodological differences among studies, there appears to be a consistent pattern in the occurrence of trauma. The patient's home has been consistently reported as the main location for sustaining dental trauma for both primary and permanent dentitions. This was closely followed by injuries in schools. It was also observed that there were an increasing number of causes. Despite this, sporting arenas, playgrounds, and roads are featured in most studies in varying proportions.

Falls are the most common activity causing trauma and account for most injuries in the primary dentition. This is unsurprising as it is typical for toddlers to crawl, stagger, and fall before being able to walk as part of their development. Although falls are featured prominently in the permanent dentition, sporting activities accounted for the majority of injuries. Other impact activities/accidents such as fights, assaults, and bicycle and motor vehicle accidents have been featured in most studies. Many of the studies reviewed showed that males experienced trauma more frequently than females in the permanent dentition; males outnumber females in sustaining trauma by a ratio ranging from 1.3 to 2.5:1, respectively. It has been postulated that males had a greater propensity toward contact sports and violent behavior [94].

Despite this, it has been noted that gender disparities were on the decline with females showing an increased participation in sports.

Traebert et al. noted that females can be exposed to the same risk factors as males which are characteristic of modern western society. Disparities in the primary dentition were generally not as significant or obvious. As falls in the primary dentition are mostly uncontrolled and given that participation in sport is by choice, it seems that gender as a risk factor is essentially related to activities undertaken. Appreciation of gender disparities is an important consideration when interpreting other epidemiological parameters. Lam et al. reported a lower age is another frequently reported risk factor where studies indicate that trauma experience was skewed toward the younger population (toddlers, children, adolescents, and young adults). The specific age(s) was another source of variation affected by local and methodological differences. Despite these differences, there is a general trend indicating toddlers who sustained injuries from involuntary falls, while adolescents experienced accidental injuries from contact sports and other impact injuries [94].

In an Australian study, Lam et al. chose to classify age in 5-year increments and found that these injuries were predominant in the 0–4-year group and the 10–14-year group. In this cohort, 92% of injuries occurred before the age of 34 years [94].

This is consistent with other studies indicating that dental trauma is skewed.

- **Assessment and Management of TDIs**

Immediate assessment of TDIs is very crucial for identifying the appropriate actions that are required to be decided by the team. In addition, immediate assessment is playing an important role for better prognosis, treatment options, and outcomes. Dentist is the first line of emergency that a patient with TDIs might visit in many cases, for instance, in the case of tooth avulsion, an immediate reimplantation will significantly improve the prognosis [95]. It was reported that the maxillary central incisors are the most common tooth liable for injuries in both primary and permanent dentitions. For primary teeth, luxation injuries were the most common oral traumatic dental injuries, while for the permanent dentition, fracture of the crown was dominating [96].

However, several studies showed lack of knowledge and general awareness regarding the emergency management of dental trauma injuries among parents [97]. Furthermore, several studies also showed lack of knowledge and awareness of the required emergency management of dental trauma injuries among other laypersons who may involve in such situations such as schoolteachers [98] and sports coaches [99]. In addition, some studies showed that the level of such awareness is varying among dental professionals themselves [100].

In order to increase such awareness, smartphone which is based on the artificial technology was proposed as an appropriate tool to act as a gateway to increase such awareness [101]. A review conducted by Djemal and Singh in 2016 has found that more than seven applications are compatible to be sued with different smartphones to enhance awareness and knowledge among different populations including dentists about emergency management of dental trauma injuries [101]. Although most of the existing applications are ranging in quality, the authors suggested that with the advances of AI technology that allow animation and integration of social media, the future apps should continue to provide good quality, evidence-based, and validated information [101].

To enhance knowledge of traumatic dental injuries, several knowledge-based systems (KBS) that are based on the technology of artificial intelligence have been proposed [102]. These AI-based software have been suggested to be used to enhance immediate assessment, diagnosis, and decision-making in case of emergency traumatized dental injuries [96].

Oral traumatic dental injuries should be treated as an emergency dental situation. One of the most important issues that affect the successful treatment of TDIs is the immediate behaviors of the patient and the persons who are present in the site of accident as well. AI-based technology that allows remote communication between patient and dentists such as tele-assistant can be very helpful till the professional visit can take place [103].

According to the American College of Surgeons, a clear and systematic protocol should be applied to any traumatized patient including first and rapid survey to ensure vital functions such as maintenance of airway with cervical spine control (A), ensuring breathing and ventilation (B), controlling circulation with hemorrhage (C), checking any disability (neurological status-D), and complete examination of the patient (E) [104]. After stabilization of the patient, a second survey can be carried out to evaluate injuries and traumatized tissues including infection control, control pain, and stabilization of fractures and to provide patient with supportive treatment. Therefore, applying the ABCDE protocol with proper diagnosis for any individuals with traumatic dental injuries is very critical and essential for correct treatment and good prognosis. Recently, there are many studies and calls for applying smart robotics with machine learning technology to act as dental assistant in order to make the process of assessing dental emergencies more rapid and accurate [103]. These robotic dental assistants will help to check vital signs of the patient quickly, in addition to other tasks that required repeated workflows that eventually will enhance dental work in the emergency situation and will free the other human resources for social interaction that cannot be done by the robotics [103].

In several cases, patient with TDIs may need replacement of the missing teeth. AI-based technology has improved the restorative procedures such as dental implant. There are several studies which used artificial intelligence-based technology such as artificial neural network and convolutional neural network with either 3D cone-beam computed tomography (CBCT) images and/or panoramic radiographs to facilitate decision-making to improve the treatment plan, assess the quality of osteointegration, and measure the peri-implant bone loss [105].

- **Management**

  Treatment of dental trauma varies according to the type of injury involved:

  - Fracture
  - Avulsion
  - Luxation (tooth displacement)

Tetanus booster and antibiotics should be administered whenever a dental injury is at risk for infection. Arrangements should be made for prompt follow-up with a dentist or an oral and maxillofacial surgeon.

Dental fractures may be classified as follows:

- Ellis class I (superficial enamel only)—No emergency care is required; follow-up with a dentist is arranged as needed.
- Ellis class II (enamel and dentin, with sensitivity to temperature, air, and palpation)—The exposed dentin is covered, preferably with dental cement; the patient is referred to a dentist within 24 h.
- Ellis class III (enamel, dentin, and pulp; a dental emergency)—The fracture is covered with dental cement; patients receive urgent and immediate dental follow-up; topical painkillers increase the risk of infection and thus should not be applied.
- Root fractures—Depending on the location of fracture, treatment varies from splinting, RCT, and even extraction.

Principles of management for dental avulsions include the following:

- An adult tooth that is avulsed should be reimplanted in its socket as soon as possible.
- If the tooth cannot be reimplanted, it should be placed in a protective solution like HBSS, cold milk, etc.; it should never be allowed to dry.
- If the tooth has been dry for a significant period, it should be soaked in the appropriate solution (which depends on the length of the dry period).
- Some studies suggest that when a tooth has been out of the mouth for longer than 60 min, immediate reimplantation is not required, and a root canal of the tooth should be performed with the tooth outside the mouth before it is reimplanted.
- After reimplantation, any other injuries are repaired.
- In children with dental avulsions, primary teeth are never reimplanted, because reimplantation of a deciduous tooth can cause harm to the developing permanent tooth.

Luxations may be classified as follows:

- Concussion—Mild injury to the periodontal ligament, with some clinical tenderness but no movement of the tooth.
- Subluxation—More significant injury to the periodontal ligament, with clinical tenderness and movement of the tooth.
- Extrusion—Partial removal of a tooth from its socket.

- Lateral luxation—Lateral displacement of a tooth at an angle, with possible fracture of the alveolar bone as well.
- Intrusion—Impaction of a tooth into its socket in the fractured alveolar bone Treatment of luxations includes the following:
- Concussion and subluxation—A soft diet, administration of nonsteroidal anti-inflammatory drugs (NSAIDs), and referral to a dentist; subluxation is a more significant injury and is more often associated with pulpal necrosis.
- Extrusion—Restoration of the tooth to its original position and splinting.
- Lateral luxation—Repositioning of the tooth, often made more difficult by a fractured alveolar bone, and splinting, done by a general practitioner only if the alveolar bone fracture is minimal and done by a dentist or an oral and maxillofacial surgeon if the fracture is more extensive.
- Intrusion—Usually, referral to a dentist within 24 hours is indicated.

Associated injuries to the maxillofacial bones may be classified as follows:

- Le Fort I—Transverse fracture separating the body of the maxilla from the lower portion of the pterygoid plate and nasal septum.
- Le Fort II—Pyramidal fracture of the central maxilla and palate; facial tugging moves the nose but not the eyes.
- Le Fort III (i.e., craniofacial disjunction)—Facial skeleton completely separated from the skull, with the fracture extending through the frontozygomatic suture lines and through the orbit, the base of the nose, and the ethmoid; on physical examination, the entire face shifts with tugging [106].

The image below depicts the Le Fort classification of maxillary fractures (Fig. 3.3).

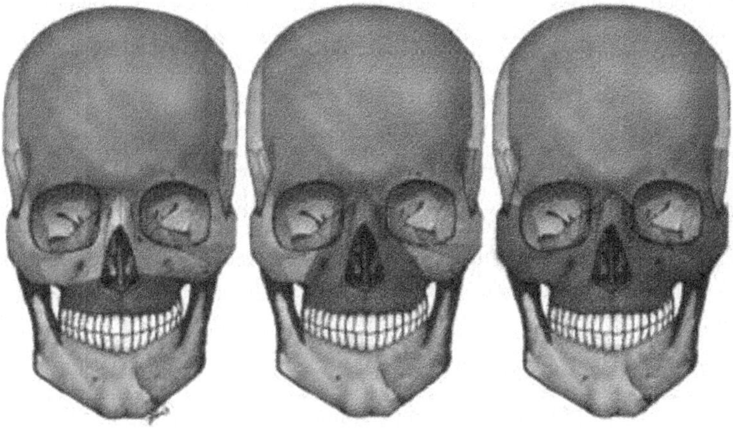

Fig. 3.3 Le Fort I, II, and III maxillary fractures. (Image source [106])

3.2.6 Noma (Cancrum Oris)

Cancrum oris or Noma is a fatal infection of the mouth that mostly affects children between the ages of 1 and 16, with a peak incidence at ages 1 to 4. It destroys soft tissues and bones of the oral and para-oral structures. It mostly affects children suffering from malnutrition, affected by infectious disease, living in extreme poverty with poor oral hygiene, and/or with weakened immune systems [4].

Noma is mostly found in sub-Saharan Africa, although cases have also been reported in Latin America and Asia. The word Noma is derived from the Greek: to "devour" that carries in one of its meaning "eat greediness" which describe the aggressiveness of the diseases that destroys the mouth and the face. Noma has many alternative names such as orofacial gangrene, cancrum, or necrotizing ulcerative gingivitis that leads to severe orofacial disfigurement and usually affects children between 2 and 6 years [107]. Noma usually starts as gingivitis that, due to its neglection, develops into gingival necrosis and if not treated the infection will spread to underlying jawbone. Eventually, infected facial region develops swelling and subsequently necrotizes, leading to destruction of soft and hard facial tissues to leave severe disfigurement [108]. Untreated Noma has an estimated mortality rate of 90% [109].

In 1998, WHO estimated that there were 140,000 new cases of Noma annually. Without treatment, Noma is fatal in 90% of cases. Survivors suffer from severe facial disfigurement, have difficulty speaking and eating, face social stigma, and require complex surgery and rehabilitation. Where Noma is detected at an early stage, its progression can be rapidly halted, through basic hygiene, antibiotics, and improved nutrition [4, 110].

- **Medical History**

Noma is an old companion of humankind. Described by classical and medieval authors, the disease was common in Europe and the United States for centuries. In 1649, Noma was included in the first book about neglected diseases, *Observationes Medicae de Affectibus Omissis*, by Arnoldus Bootius. By the end of the nineteenth century, Noma gradually disappeared from European and US hospitals due to increasing improvements in the welfare of the population. In the rare Noma cases that crossed the paths of bacteriologists in the twentieth century, no conclusive findings about the causative microorganisms were made until Stewart concluded in 1912 that Noma was not a specific infection, but rather an opportunistic one caused by normal oral flora. Shortly after the introduction of sulfonamides and penicillin in the 1940s, it appeared that treatment with antimicrobial drugs reduced the mortality of Noma from around 85% to approximately 15%. By contrast, a clear concept with regard to reconstructive Noma surgery was developed only 50 years ago [110].

- **Etiological Considerations**

Noma has a multifactorial etiology. A prerequisite is malnutrition, often related to extreme poverty, but other factors are concomitant diseases and poor oral hygiene resulting in gingivitis. Malnutrition is closely correlated with immunity, which may lead to a nutritionally acquired immune deficiency syndrome. This condition is particularly prevalent in children who were preterm and low-birth-weight babies. Depending on the region in Africa, these infants represent up to 25% of births. The age of the onset of Noma corresponds nutritionally to a period of vulnerability coinciding with the period of weaning, with underweight infants particularly at risk. Importantly, weaning corresponds also to the age of the onset of debilitating and immunosuppressive diseases, such as the first malaria crisis or measles.

Social factors play a role in the onset of Noma, particularly in large families where the mother has grand multiparity and an inadequate nutritional status. The link between the number of past pregnancies and chronic malnutrition in children with Noma suggests that it could be related to maternal malnutrition during pregnancy. This may increase the risk for prematurity or low-birth-weight infants, thus promoting a vicious cycle of repetitive infections and chronic malnutrition and opening the door for Noma onset. Various diseases have been described in association with Noma, such as malaria, typhus, measles, chickenpox, tuberculosis, and HIV infection. Measles and malaria are the most frequently reported illnesses that precede Noma. These diseases often occur during the weaning period and have serious immunosuppressive effects.

Insufficient oral hygiene can facilitate the onset of a necrotizing gingivitis characterized by the presence of some periodontal pathogens and sometimes resulting in the development of Noma [110].

- **Clinical Signs Preceding Noma**

Noma does not start as a necrotizing process. It is preceded by a small intraoral ulcer, by an aphthous lesion, or, frequently, by acute necrotizing gingivitis (ANG). ANG is characterized by spontaneous bleeding, ulceration of the gingival papillae, pain, and sometimes, grayish pseudomembranes. In Africa, there is a high prevalence of ANG in children that ranges from 15% to 60%, depending on the region and the degree of poverty. ANG is facilitated by the lack of dental hygiene, but there is also evidence that malnutrition alone can lead to changes in the oral microflora and to ANG. In general, ANG can be treated by improving oral hygiene, but if the child is undernourished and dental hygiene with follow-up cannot be achieved, antibiotics are recommended. Without treatment, ANG may evolve into a necrotizing stomatitis and result in the destruction of the attached gingival mucosa, the surrounding oral mucosa, and the underlying bones. This stage requires antibiotic treatment. If no treatment is undertaken, the risk of progression toward Noma is very high [110].

Acute Noma: Stage of Edema and Halitosis

The starting point of Noma is defined when facial edema appears in addition to intraoral necrotizing stomatitis, accompanied by a typical halitosis often considered as pathognomonic. This stage is short and lasts only a few days [110].

Acute Noma: Stage of Necrosis
Following the appearance of necrotizing stomatitis and facial edema, a necrotizing infection extends rapidly within a few days into the intraoral mucosa, the facial muscles, the skin, the maxilla, and the mandible. A bluish discoloration of the skin indicates underlying necrosis coming to the surface. A peculiarity of this gangrene is that it appears to have a self-limiting character ending in a well-demarcated necrosis. On some occasions, the body appears to be able to resist and halt the expansion of the gangrene at a certain stage. Interestingly, some children do not receive treatment and develop relatively small lesions, while others experience huge facial destruction despite appropriate medical treatment. This may be due to differences in the degree of impairment of their immune systems [110].

Acute Noma: Stage of Sloughs and Healing
After demarcation of the gangrene, the necrotic tissue starts to slough. At this stage, many patients die due to sepsis. If they do survive and the body has eliminated most necrotic tissue by sloughing, suppuration, or sequestration, signs of wound healing appear. During this stage, granulation tissue forms, wound contracture occurs, and both mucosa and epithelium start to grow from the margins of the wound over the granulating surface. Depending on the tissue defect and the health of the patient, this healing process may take weeks or many months. The wound healing process may lead to intraoral constricting bands hampering normal mouth opening (trismus) and, in severe cases, to fibrous or even bony ankylosis of the temporomandibular joint. The dramatic result of this condition is the fact that it will impair the nutrition of children who are already undernourished [110].

- **Noma Sequelae**

Only approximately 15% of children survive acute Noma. Most survivors present with facial deformities and trismus or ankylosis of the mandible, resulting in eating problems, oral incontinence, speech difficulties, and social isolation. At a later age, these contractures often lead to growth disturbances and result in further facial disfigurement and functional impairment. The psychological impact of surviving Noma can be easily understood, but it has been rarely studied [110].

- **Classification**

Noma can be classified using mainly two systems, the first system introduced by Marck et al. (NOITULP) [111] and the second system introduced by Montandon et al. (Montandon) [112]. Montandon classification was based on the severity of the defect and the surgical approach for treatment and replacing the defects of the face as the main tool for classification of the condition. Although this method of classification was validated by the WHO in 1994, it lacks the consistency and is not a quantified method and errors can take place [109].

The NOITULP classification is another method that is relying on combination involvement of different anatomical structure such as the nose, lip, cheek, mandible, and maxilla. The description of the letters of NOITULP is as follows: N, "nose"; O, "outer cheek"; I, "inner cheek"; T, "trismus"; U, "upper lip"; L, "lower lip"; and P, "particularities." The combination of involvement and severity of such anatomical landmarks is used to rate the condition from 0 to 4.

According to NOITULP classification, Noma can be classified into four types: Type I includes features of a localized lip damage, commissure, or cheek defect that is lined by local tissues and covered with a single flap; Type II includes an upper lip and nose amputation; Type III presents with a lower lip and mandible amputation, and Type IV includes large defects involving the lips, cheek, palate, maxillary bone, and orbital floor [109].

- **Preventive Measures**

Primary prevention of Noma can be achieved by economic development, but only if this development ensures that parents can feed their children adequately. Food security programs may be less desirable, but they are effective. However, these preventive measures are political and public health issues. Primary medical prevention of Noma consists of measles vaccination programs and the prevention and treatment of concomitant diseases, such as HIV and malaria. Secondary prevention includes the detection and treatment before visible symptoms are difficult to treat and requires surveillance programs in areas of famine and poverty where limited resources are already stretched to the limit by other health priorities.

Tertiary prevention of the disease consists of methods to reduce the negative impact of symptomatic disease, such as disability or death, through treatment and rehabilitation.

Noma is not a common disease, but typically occurs with other neglected diseases and malnutrition. Noma should not be targeted alone, in contrast with vertical programs aiming to eradicate specific health conditions, such as the nearly successful eradication of guinea worm infection. Rather, Noma should be included in neglected disease, poverty, malnutrition, and health education programs [110].

- **Treatment**

The treatment is usually by surgical intervention and facial construction; however, many complications can occur such as infection, partial flap necrosis, total flap loss and necrosis, bleeding/hematoma, donor site dehiscence, and recurrent fistula [109].

Surgical treatment may require in some severe cases prosthesis replacement to recover function and ethics. Conventionally, fabrication of soft tissue prosthesis requires following time-consuming protocol that contains several technical steps including taking impression of the area of facial defect, creating color-matched silicon molds, and converting these molds into a product [113]. However, applying different artificial intelligence-based technology in this field results in great success, saving time with great accuracy and patient satisfaction. This technology includes 3D scanning and digital impression, computer-aided design (CAD), and 3D printing technologies [114].

Several recent studies that used the advances of artificial intelligence technology demonstrated a promising result to improve the prosthetic replacement. For example, a recent study was conducted by Mine et al., in 2020, who used two types of machine learning algorithms which are ANN-based deep learning and the random forest algorithm to determine the best pigment that can match skin of the patient [115]. The study found that the deep ANN approach produced superior predictive results with respect to color of matching [115].

Conclusion

Noma is a noncontagious infectious disease with a relatively high burden of disease and should be part of neglected tropical disease programs. The neglect of Noma is a major humanitarian concern that requires the attention of national and international organizations. Noma is a biological indicator of extreme poverty, malnutrition, and human rights violations affecting the most vulnerable children. The vicious cycle of Noma neglect begins with WHO and continues without awareness or monitoring, which keeps the disease unknown throughout the world. Therefore, Noma should be on the WHO list of neglected tropical diseases. Wherever Noma is found, primary health care is needed to improve nutrition, immunizations, exclusive breastfeeding, hygiene, sanitation, and dental care [110].

3.2.7 Cleft Lip and Palate

Clefts of the lip or palate affect more than 1 in 1000 newborns worldwide. Genetic predisposition is a major cause. However, poor maternal nutrition, tobacco consumption, alcohol use, and obesity during pregnancy also play a role. In low-income settings, there is a high mortality rate in the neonatal period. If lip and palate clefts are properly treated by surgery, complete rehabilitation is possible [4].

More than four million children are born with birth defects worldwide every year. Craniofacial anomalies comprise a large fraction of all human birth defects, less frequent only than congenital heart disorders and clubfoot. Cleft lip with or without palate (CL/P) is the most common craniofacial birth defect with an estimated quarter of a million affected babies born each year in the world. This malformation shows considerable variation across geographic regions and ethnic groups and has significant medical, psychological, social, and economic ramifications. It is a costly public health problem with an average lifetime treatment cost per child in the United States estimated to be roughly $101,000 [116].

The World Health Organization (WHO) and most cleft organizations across the globe recommend interdisciplinary care by a team of specialists. In reality, however, surgical and nonsurgical treatment is often fragmented and dictated by socioeconomic factors and access to medical facilities. In developing countries, particularly in rural areas, care is often neglected due to social beliefs and lack of awareness, or initiated late due to restricted resources and inadequate access. The delay in treatment and intermittent care by local or overseas cleft mission surgeons, combined with incomplete follow-up, results in poor outcomes with unnecessary complications. More recently, some humanitarian nonprofit organizations supporting cleft care have changed their aid philosophy.

The WHO initiative for collaborative craniofacial anomalies research has identified areas of uncertainty in clinical care, and efforts are being made to conduct trials with sufficiently large samples of patients to provide evidence for treatment strategies. Initial research efforts have focused on addressing surgical, anesthetic, and nursing care for patients with craniofacial anomalies in developing countries. Surgical techniques for repair of various cleft subtypes and correction of velopharyngeal insufficiency are being evaluated. Adjunctive services such as use of prophylactic ventilation tubes, presurgical orthopedics, psychological counseling, speech therapy, and feeding interventions before and after surgery are also being monitored and assessed. An international database of craniofacial anomalies has been established to improve answers to questions relevant to individuals with cleft and craniofacial anomalies, their families, and health-care providers [116].

- **Etiology**

CP is more common in females and more often associated with other developmental anomalies. Environmental factors that include maternal cigarette smoking, alcohol consumption, and multivitamin use are the three factors most considered with regard to the risks of isolated cleft lip and palate. These two important domains, environmental and genetic, are intersecting together and affecting each other when it comes to the cleft lip and cleft palate [117]. The result in the literature is suggesting a possible link between maternal alcohol consumption and markers in chromosome 9 in cases of isolated cleft palate. So, it was suggested that consuming alcoholic drinks during the first trimester of pregnancy increases the risk of oral clefts in the offspring [118]. Furthermore, it appears that children carrying specific genetic variation in ADH1C (alcohol dehydrogenase 1C) are at higher risks to have oral clefts if their mothers were alcohol drinkers. Similarly, there is also a possible association between maternal cigarette smoking and markers in TBK1 (TANK binding kinase 1) on chromosome 12 and ZNF236 (zinc finger protein 236) on chromosome 18 [119]. In addition, the literature demonstrated an inverse relationship between the use of maternal multivitamin and the risk for cleft and palate, i.e., the more multivitamin use, the less chance for isolated cleft palate. There are strong evidence suggesting a strong interaction between the two genetic molecules IRF6 and ZNF533 and maternal vitamin use as decreasing the susceptibility to isolated cleft lip and palate [120].

Clefts are referred to as non-syndromic and syndromic, based on their association with other anomalies. About 50% of CP and 10% of CL/P are associated with a syndrome. Some common syndromes associated with cleft lip and palate include Van der Woude syndrome, Treacher Collins syndrome, Down syndrome, orofacial digital syndrome, Opitz syndrome, craniofacial microsomia, and fetal alcohol syndrome. Nearly half of the syndromic cleft palate presentations are associated with the triad of micrognathia, glossoptosis, and airway obstruction (Pierre Robin sequence). The most common syndromic presentations of this triad are Stickler's syndrome, accounting for 25%, and velo-cardio-facial (VCF) syndrome, accounting for 15% of all syndromic cleft palate individuals.

Non-syndromic CLP is a complex trait with multifactorial etiology, resulting from gene-gene and gene-environmental interactions. Identification of key genes contributing to the genesis of orofacial clefts will help in early diagnosis, disease prevention, or possibly developing adjunctive therapies. The most recent estimates suggest that anywhere from 3 to 14 genes contribute to cleft lip and palate. Important contributors to CL/P are variants of interferon regulatory growth factor 6 (IRF 6) gene, whose function is related to the formation of connective tissue. Mutations in IRF6 lead to Van der Woude and popliteal pterygium syndromes.

Aberrant transforming growth factor beta-3 (TGF-β3) signaling plays a role in the pathogenesis of cleft palate. Environmental factors that contribute to the etiology of facial clefting disorders include cigarette smoking, folic acid deficiency during the periconceptional period, and maternal exposure to alcohol and teratogenic medications such as retinoids, corticosteroids, and anticonvulsants (phenytoin and valproic acid). Consanguineous marriages, maternal diabetes, and obesity have also been linked to an increased risk of orofacial clefts. Less consistent associations have been found between clefts and maternal viral infections such as rubella and varicella [116].

- **Embryology**

The embryologic development of the face begins at 4 weeks after conception from the neural crest ectomesenchyme that forms five prominences, the frontonasal process, and paired maxillary and mandibular processes surrounding a central depression. During the fifth and sixth weeks of embryonic development, bilateral maxillary processes derived from first brachial arch fuse with the medial nasal process to form the upper lip, alveolus, and the primary palate [116] (Fig. 3.4).

The lateral nasal process forms the alar structures of the nose. The lower lip and jaw are formed by the mandibular processes. This process of formation of the face is the consequence of a cascade of processes that involve cell proliferation, cell differentiation, cell adhesion, and apoptosis. Failure or error in any of these cellular processes that lead to fusion of the medial nasal process with the lateral nasal and maxillary process can cause orofacial clefts.

- **Classification**

In order to standardize documentation and communicate effectively, various types of classification systems have been described.

The early Veau classification included groups 1–4 with increasing severity of clefting [60]:

- Group 1—cleft of the soft palate
- Group 2—cleft of the hard and soft palate up to incisive foramen
- Group 3—complete unilateral cleft lip and palate
- Group 4—complete bilateral cleft lip and palate

However, this classification is not always adequate to document the variations. The more sophisticated schematic diagrams, such as the one described by Kernahan and Stark, have been used recently [116].

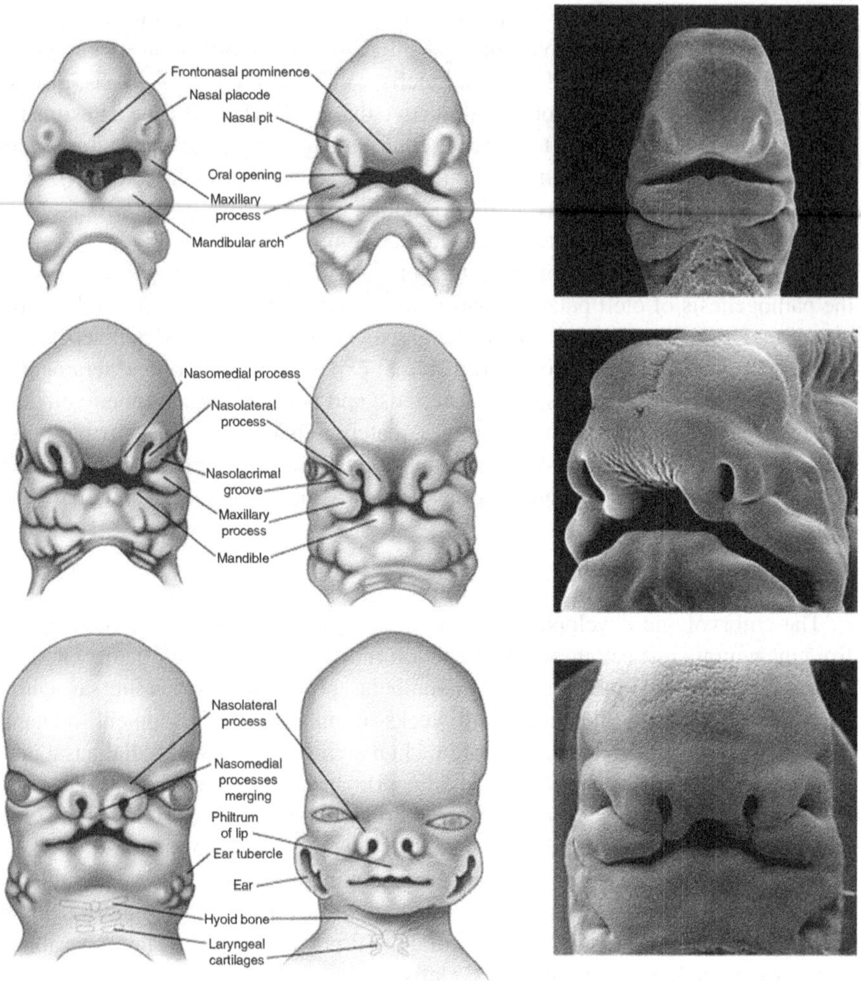

Fig. 3.4 Development of the nose and face. (Image source [121])

Berkowitz used a simple classification for labio-palatine clefts:

1. Clefts of lip and alveolus
2. Clefts of primary (including lip) and secondary palate
3. Clefts of secondary palate only
4. Submucous cleft [61, 62] (Fig. 3.5)

- **Diagnosis**

Interdisciplinary team care begins with prenatal diagnosis and parental counseling. With the advent of sophisticated high-resolution three-dimensional (3D) ultrasonography and genetic tests for screening of birth defects, intrauterine diagnosis of

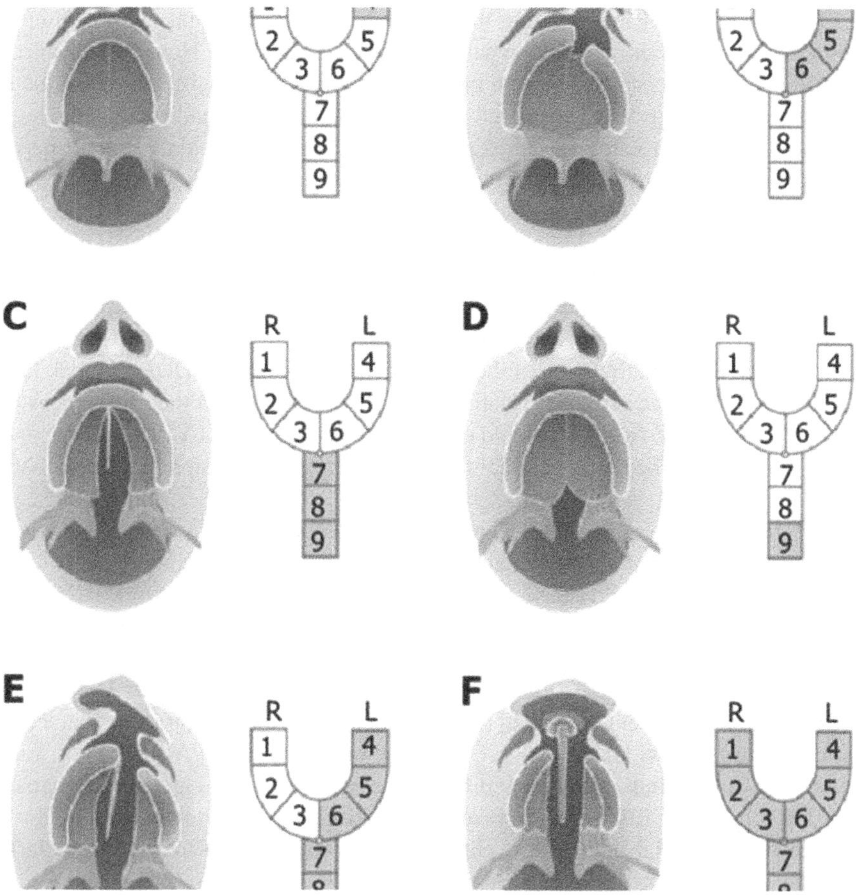

Fig. 3.5 Kernahan's classification

cleft lip is possible. Early diagnosis of a cleft of the lip should alert the obstetrician of the possibility of other malformations that may require further investigations.

While early diagnosis may help parents to be better prepared, the advent of such a capability raises both ethical and psychological issues, such as dilemma of termination of birth. Physicians and surgeons must inform parents that CLP in the absence of other major systemic anomalies is a treatable non-life-threatening condition. The cleft team also can discuss feeding issues and timing of lip and palate surgery and help establish contact with support groups for the family.

Premaxillary protrusion is an important clue to the presence of cleft lip and cleft palate and may be more conspicuous than the cleft itself. The presence of a paranasal echogenic mass favors the presence of bilateral cleft lip and cleft palate. Clefts of palate alone are rarely visualized on ultrasound. The majority of the cases of orofacial clefts are detected antenatally [122].

The challenges of investigating the influence of environmental factors on cleft susceptibility are mainly related to data collection and analysis. However, advances in artificial intelligences resulted in increasing medical data digitization and documentation. These advances improved generation, maintaining and processing large amount of data that can be used to provide the clinicians not only diagnostic or predictive data but also help improve decision-making. Furthermore, advances in the technology of the artificial intelligences including different software specially for molecular medicine including DNA sequencing, RNA sequencing, and bioinformatics have revolutionized the data collection and information analysis to study the impact of the environmental factors on the gene expression. For example, a very recent study, conducted by Young et al., in 2021, tries to examine the epigenetic effect on the DNA methylation of the monozygotic (MZ) twins' DNA as a risk factor of non-syndromic orofacial cleating [123]. The study found that differences in certain genes in MZ twin pairs could explain the discordant NSCLP phenotype and show the effect of the environmental factor on the gene expression in patients with NSCLP [123].

Artificial intelligence-based technology has been used successfully to not just predict risk factors but also to diagnose and identify CL/P in patients. A study conducted by Agarwal et al., in 2018, using convolutional neural network (CNN) to analyze camera digital image succeeded in diagnosing, identifying, and classifying cleft lip and palate in infants [124]. Two studies conducted by the same authors, Alam and Alfawzan, in 2020 using AI-based software analyzed the radiographic characteristics of patients with oral clefts and compared the radiographic characteristic to normal individuals [125, 126]. They showed that using AI-based software was successful to find a significant difference related to skeletal and dental characteristics related to CL/P between normal individuals and individuals with CL/P.

Recently, artificial intelligence played an important role in treating oral clefts helping the clinicians for the appropriate surgical decision minimizing the errors and variations in the surgical outcomes due to different clinicians' experiences. A recent study conducted by Li et al., in 2019, used a novel robotic surgery assistant that is based on deep learning machines to analyze frontal photographs of the infants with oral clefts in order to identify the surgical markers and incisions during surgical corrections of the clefts [127]. However, other two studies used AI- based technology to analyze cephalometric parameters to predict early if the infants will need orthognathic surgery later [128, 129]. Another interesting study by Schiebl, Bauer, Grill, and Loeffelbein in 2020 showed that AI-based technology can even be used before the surgery to minimize the severity of oral clefts [130]. In this study, the authors succeeded to virtually study the growth of the maxillary arch with clefts and by using the technology of 3D printing to design and fabricate successive plates to close the gaps due to oral clefts. This approach succeeded to minimize the severity of cleft lip and palate in infants who are required nasoalveolar molding [130].

- **Interdisciplinary Care of the Cleft Patient** [131]

Prenatal
Diagnosis and parental counseling

0–6 months
General assessment for associated anomalies
ENT evaluation—breathing, feeding, swallowing, and hearing
Presurgical orthopedics (0–3 months)
Primary lip repair (3–4 months)

6 months–2 years
Speech and oral sensory motor assessment Grommets/ear tubes (as needed)
Primary palate repair (9–12 months)

Preschool: 3–5 years
Dental care
Speech assessment and therapy (continue as needed)
Assess need for lip revision

Childhood: 6–12 years
Correction of velopharyngeal dysfunction (as needed)
Orthodontic treatment—phase I
Alveolar cleft repair (8–11 years)

Adolescence: 13–18 years
Orthodontic treatment—phase II
Orthognathic surgery (if needed)—14–16 years (female)
16–18 years (male)
Revision cheilo-rhinoplasty
Replacement of missing teeth (as needed)

Conclusion
The repair of cleft lip and palate is both challenging and rewarding. Most of the existing literature is practice-centered with retrospective data. Furthermore, there is a shift toward patient-reported outcomes regarding satisfaction and quality of life. Cleft care has evolved steadily over the past decade and research has advanced our understanding of the sequelae of these anomalies and the implications of various treatment options.

3.3 Overview of Oral Manifestations of Systemic Disease

On examination, the oral cavity may exhibit manifestations of underlying systemic disease and serve as an indicator of overall health and allow for early diagnosis and treatment. Systemic diseases with oral findings include autoimmune, hematologic, endocrine, and neoplastic processes. Autoimmune disease may manifest as oral ulcerations, changes in the salivary and parotid glands, and changes in the tongue. Patients with hematologic illnesses may present with gingival bleeding or tongue changes such as glossitis, depending on the etiology. Oral changes associated with endocrine illness are variable and depend on the underlying condition. Neoplastic changes include metastatic lesions to the bony and soft tissues of the oral cavity. Patients with chronic diseases such as gastroesophageal reflux and eating disorders may present with dental erosions that cause oral pain or halitosis. In the pediatric population, oral changes can be related to rare cancers, such as Langerhans cell histiocytosis, or infectious etiologies, such as Kawasaki disease. In both adults and pediatric patients, poor oral health has been linked to poorer health outcomes overall. Thorough history taking and physical examination by dentists may aid in determining the underlying etiology of oral changes and allow for earlier intervention by medical colleagues [132].

It has been well known for a long time that the oral cavity acts as the diagnostic zone of the human body that contributes to a great extent in detection of several local and/or systemic diseases [133]. The US Surgeon General's report Oral Health in America in 2000 highlighted the importance of oral examination in diagnosing immunologic diseases, endocrinopathies, hematologic conditions, systemic infections, and nutritional disorders [134].

3.3.1 Oral Mucosal Manifestations

- **Autoimmune Diseases: Sjogren's Syndrome**

Sjogren's syndrome (SS) is an autoimmune condition predominantly seen in women aged 50 years or older, affecting the major salivary glands (parotid gland) with female is to male ratio as 9:1 [135]. Sjogren's syndrome (SS) is classified into two: primary Sjogren's comprising of xerophthalmia and xerostomia and secondary Sjogren's associated with rheumatoid arthritis or systemic lupus erythematosus [136]. The most observed oral lesions in patients diagnosed with SS were found to be in association with xerostomia: angular cheilitis, atrophic glossitis, fungal infestation with *Candida albicans*, recurrent ulcerations, fissuration of the tongue, and increased susceptibility to dental caries [137]. SS is reported to have a malignant transformation rate of 4.3% [137], recognizing the oral manifestations at an early stage can prevent the formation of low-grade marginal zone lymphoma (MALT), diffuse B-cell lymphoma (DBCL), or lymphoplasmacytoid lymphoma [137].

- **Pemphigus Vulgaris**

Pemphigus vulgaris (PV) is a chronic autoimmune mucocutaneous disorder which affects patients in the fourth and sixth decade of life with female predominance. In PV IgG autoantibodies are directed against glycoproteins, desmoglein 1 (Dsg 1), and desmoglein 3 (Dsg 3) present in the desmosomes of epithelial tissue leading to acantholysis and concomitant occurrence of intraepithelial vesicles and bullae [138]. Oral lesions precede skin lesions and are the earliest manifestation of the disease in 50–90% of the cases [139]. In the early stages of the disease, blisters are predominantly seen in relation to the buccal mucosa, lower lip, gingiva, ventral tongue, and soft palate which burst leaving behind eroded or ulcerated areas followed by desquamative gingivitis observed in the advanced stages of the disease [138].

- **Hematologic Diseases: Iron Deficiency Anemia**

Iron deficiency anemia (IDA) is the most common type of anemia where the hemoglobin content of blood is lower than the normal. It is seen particularly among preschool children and women in developing countries [140]. Iron deficiency anemia could occur due to improper dietary intake of folic acid, iron, and vitamin B12 [141]. A few leading oral manifestations of IDA include pallor of the oral mucosa, dry mouth, burning sensation, atrophic glossitis, angular cheilitis, fissured tongue, oral lichen planus, oral pigmentations, and recurrent oral ulcerations [142]. According to WHO, the key to reduce the incidence of anemia is timely screening and the availability of nutrient supplements for the treatment of anemic women [143].

- **Pernicious Anemia**

Pernicious anemia (PA) is a rare autoimmune disorder characterized by the absence of intrinsic factor in the stomach leading to the impairment of vitamin B12 absorption [144]. Several oral manifestations such as glossitis, glossodynia, recurrent ulcers, cheilitis, dysgeusia, lingual paresthesia, and burning sensation are observed [145]. One needs to understand that not all patients who are diagnosed with vitamin B12 deficiency will develop PA [145].

- **Leukemia**

Leukemia is a true malignant neoplasm characterized by progressive overproduction of immature white blood cells in the circulating blood that can be presented as acute or chronic conditions [146]. Presence of oral manifestations in leukemic patients may indicate an initial evidence or recurrence of the disease. Oral manifestations can be seen in both acute and chronic leukemia [147]. One of the earliest oral manifestations seen in acute monocytic, lymphocytic, and myelocytic leukemia is generalized gingival enlargement [147]. Other oral manifestations such as ulcers, gingival bleeding, ecchymosis, and bluish or pale oral mucosal changes accompanied with tissue necrosis are also observed [148].

- **Langerhans Cell Histiocytosis (Histiocytosis X)**

Langerhans cell histiocytosis (LCH) is a rare disorder predominantly seen in males and characterized by intense and abnormal proliferation of bone marrow-derived histiocytes (Langerhans cells) [149]. Oral manifestations such as ulcerations, gingival bleeding, odontalgia, dental hypermobility, and premature loss of teeth are commonly seen in patients diagnosed with LCH [150]. The most common site involved is the hard palate mucosa [150]. LCH should always be considered as a differential diagnosis for advanced periodontal diseases [151].

- **Metabolic Disorders: Diabetes Mellitus**

Diabetes mellitus (DM) is a chronic metabolic disorder caused due to the deficiency of insulin secretion or resistance to insulin or both and is characterized by hyperglycemia [152]. According to transversal and longitudinal studies, DM is associated with periodontal disease-causing bacteremia and systemic inflammation [153]. Patients with uncontrolled glycemic index also demonstrate a higher prevalence rate of periapical lesions, xerostomia, dental caries, oral lichen planus, geographic tongue, and taste disturbances. A few studies enlist the association between DM and oral candidiasis which is still a controversy [153–155], although fungal infections such as mucormycosis are well documented [155].

It is very clear that there are similarities and overlaps between several oral manifestations due to systemic diseases. For example, aphthous ulcer can occur due to multiple factors and reasons such as genetic backgrounds and dietary intake, and also it can follow several systemic conditions. Therefore, diagnosis of such multifactorial conditions by excluding other factors is very important for formulating the treatment plan and improving the treatment outcome. Recently, AI-based technology such as artificial neural networks (ANNs) started to play an important role for diagnosis such as multifactorial oral lesions, for example, a study conducted by Dar-Odeh et al., in 2010, who used artificial neural networks (ANN) [156]. In this study, the authors used input data from 86 participants including predisposing factors to construct and train the artificial neural networks' machine. The study showed that ANNs succeeded to accurately predict recurrent aphthous ulcers identifying the most important factors that can be related to aphthous ulceration including gender, hemoglobin, serum vitamin B12, serum ferritin, red cell folate, salivary candida colony count, frequency of tooth brushing, and the number of fruits or vegetables consumed daily [156].

3.4 Global Epidemiological Overview of Oral Diseases

Globally, oral diseases are the most prevalent category of diseases that have an adverse impact on life of those whom affected causing major economic and health burdens [157]. Worldwide, oral diseases are considered and representing a major public health burden; however, it is frequently neglected till date. For example, Noma, which is an aggressive ulcerative oral disease due to neglection, has an incidence around 30,000–140,000 of new cases per year, globally [109].

Interestingly, it has been observed that 90% of the world's population at some point in their life have been affected by some forms of oral diseases [158]. In one of its reports published in 2005, WHO emphasized that oral diseases persisted particularly in the underprivileged groups in both developed and developing countries despite the advances in treatment modalities [159]. It is imperative to understand that oral health is integral to general health which has been proven time and again with evidence [159].

Dental caries (tooth decay), periodontal (gum) diseases, and oral cancers have been considered historically as the key clinical conditions of global public health [158, 160]. According to the data extracted from Global Burden of Diseases (GBD) in 2016, an average of 45.6% increase in dental caries (tooth decay), periodontal (gum) diseases, and oral cancers was observed from 1990 to 2010 [158]. Global epidemiological data in accordance with GBD in 2015 reported around 3.5 billion people worldwide who are affected with dental conditions predominantly severe periodontal diseases, untreated dental caries, and edentulism. On the contrary in 2018, oral cavity cancers were among the top 15 common cancers as per the International Agency for Research on Cancer (IARC) [157]. Last on the list is oro-dental trauma due to the unavailability of reliable data in most of the developing countries [160]. In addition, cleft lip and cleft palate have been ranked the second most common orofacial abnormalities at birth that add more challenges and present as a major oral health condition contributing to the global burden of oral disease that require a complete rehabilitation treatment [161].

It is now evident that oral disorders are highly prevalent and that a dental epidemiologic transition is underway at the global level. The sizable burden of oral disorders (measured as disability-adjusted life years (DALYs)) and their socioeconomic impact make them an important global public health issue. Improving our understanding of the contribution of behavioral and physiologic risk factors, social and economic determinants, and health delivery systems to oral health and well-being at the population level may not be an easy task, but untangling this complex web will help reduce disease burden and enhance life. Although there are many challenges affecting oral health research, there are opportunities. We should not forget the "3.5 billion" statistic; we should remember that we have a responsibility to continue to learn, to improve, and to measure on [162].

References

1. Nayyar N, Ojcius DM, Dugoni AA (2020) The role of medicine and technology in shaping the future of oral health. J Calif Dent Assoc 48(3):127–130
2. Ahmed N, Abbasi MS, Zuberi F, Qamar W, Halim MSB, Maqsood A, Alam MK (2021) Artificial intelligence techniques: analysis, application, and outcome in dentistry – a systematic review. Biomed Res Int 2021:9751564. https://doi.org/10.1155/2021/9751564
3. Hung M, Park J, Hon ES, Bounsanga J, Moazzami S, Ruiz-Negron B, Wang D (2020) Artificial intelligence in dentistry: harnessing big data to predict oral cancer survival. World J Clin Oncol 11(11):918–934. https://doi.org/10.5306/wjco.v11.i11.918
4. World Health Organisation (2022 Mar 15) Oral health. https://www.who.int/news-room/fact-sheets/detail/oral-health
5. Marcenes W, Kassebaum NJ, Bernabé E, Flaxman A, Naghavi M, Lopez A, Murray CJL (2013) Global burden of oral conditions in 1990–2010: a systematic analysis. J Dent Res 92(7):592–597. https://doi.org/10.1177/0022034513490168
6. Abid A, Maatouk F, Berrezouga L, Azodo C, Uti O, El-Shamy H, Oginni A (2015) Prevalence and severity of oral diseases in the Africa and Middle East region. Adv Dent Res 27(1):10–17. https://doi.org/10.1177/0022034515582062
7. Yap AU (2017) Oral health equals total health: a brief review. Literature review. J Dent Indones 24(2):59–62. https://doi.org/10.14693/jdi.v24i2.1122. https://www.researchgate.net/publication/319919543_Oral_Health_Equals_Total_Health_A_Brief_Review/fulltext/59c1d4c2a6fdcc69b92bcdd0/Oral-Health-Equals-Total-Health-A-Brief-Review.pdf

47. Armitage GC (1999 Dec) Development of a classification system for periodontal diseases and conditions. Ann Periodontol 4(1):1–6. https://doi.org/10.1902/annals.1999.4.1.1. PMID: 10863370
48. Lang NP, Tonetti MS (2003) Periodontal risk assessment (PRA) for patients in supportive periodontal therapy (SPT). Oral Health Prev Dent 1(1):7–16
49. Monsarrat P, Bernard D, Marty M, Cecchin-Albertoni C, Doumard E, Gez L et al (2022) Systemic periodontal risk score using an innovative machine learning strategy: an observational study. J Pers Med 12(2). https://doi.org/10.3390/jpm12020217
50. Özmeric N, Kostioutchenko I, Hägler G, Frentzen M, Jervøe-Storm P-M (2008) Cone-beam computed tomography in assessment of periodontal ligament space: in vitro study on artificial tooth model. Clin Oral Investig 12(3):233–239
51. Choi J-W (2011) Assessment of panoramic radiography as a national oral examination tool: review of the literature. Imaging Sci Dent 41(1):1–6
52. Lee JH, Kim DH, Jeong SN, Choi SH (2018) Diagnosis and prediction of periodontally compromised teeth using a deep learning-based convolutional neural network algorithm. J Periodontal Implant Sci 48(2):114–123. https://doi.org/10.5051/jpis.2018.48.2.114
53. Krois J, Ekert T, Meinhold L, Golla T, Kharbot B, Wittemeier A et al (2019) Deep learning for the radiographic detection of periodontal bone loss. Sci Rep 9(1):8495. https://doi.org/10.1038/s41598-019-44839-3
54. Chang HJ, Lee SJ, Yong TH, Shin NY, Jang BG, Kim JE et al (2020) Deep learning hybrid method to automatically diagnose periodontal bone loss and stage periodontitis. Sci Rep 10(1):7531. https://doi.org/10.1038/s41598-020-64509-z
55. Liu L, Xu J, Huan Y, Zou Z, Yeh SC, Zheng LR (2020) A smart dental health-IoT platform based on intelligent hardware, deep learning, and mobile terminal. IEEE J Biomed Health Inform 24(3):898–906. https://doi.org/10.1109/JBHI.2019.2919916
56. Huang W, Wu J, Mao Y, Zhu S, Huang GF, Petritis B, Huang RP (2020) Developing a periodontal disease antibody array for the prediction of severe periodontal disease using machine learning classifiers. J Periodontol 91(2):232–243. https://doi.org/10.1002/jper.19-0173
57. Farhadian M, Shokouhi P, Torkzaban P (2020) A decision support system based on support vector machine for diagnosis of periodontal disease. BMC Res Notes 13(1):337. https://doi.org/10.1186/s13104-020-05180-5
58. Mayo Clinic. Patient care & health information. Diseases and conditions. Periodontitis. https://www.mayoclinic.org/diseases-conditions/periodontitis/diagnosis-treatment/drc-20354479
59. Mayo Clinic. Patient care & health information. Diseases and conditions. Mouth Cancer. https://www.mayoclinic.org/diseases-conditions/mouth-cancer/symptoms-causes/syc-20350997
60. Cancer Research UK (2017 Nov 29) Together we will beat cancer. https://news.cancerresearchuk.org/2017/11/29/men-twice-as-likely-to-develop-oral-cancer/
61. Johnson S (2020, Sept 1) Medically reviewed by Yamini Ranchod. Healthline. Oral cancer. https://www.healthline.com/health/oral-cancer
62. Cancer.Net, ASCO, Types of cancer – Head and neck cancer. https://www.cancer.net/cancer-types/head-and-neck-cancer/diagnosis
63. American Academy of Oral Medicine (Producer) (2019) Subject: oral cancer screening. https://www.aaom.com/clinical-practicestatement-oral-cancer-screening.
64. Khanagar SB, Naik S, Al Kheraif AA, Vishwanathaiah S, Maganur PC, Alhazmi Y et al (2021) Application and performance of artificial intelligence technology in oral cancer diagnosis and prediction of prognosis: a systematic review. Diagnostics (Basel) 11(6). https://doi.org/10.3390/diagnostics11061004
65. Ilhan B, Lin K, Guneri P, Wilder-Smith P (2020) Improving oral cancer outcomes with imaging and artificial intelligence. J Dent Res 99(3):241–248. https://doi.org/10.1177/0022034520902128
66. Sinevici N, O'Sullivan J (2016) Oral cancer: deregulated molecular events and their use as biomarkers. Oral Oncol 61:12–18. https://doi.org/10.1016/j.oraloncology.2016.07.013

67. Sankaranarayanan R, Ramadas K, Thomas G, Muwonge R, Thara S, Mathew B, Rajan B (2005) Effect of screening on oral cancer mortality in Kerala, India: a cluster-randomised controlled trial. Lancet 365(9475):1927–1933. https://doi.org/10.1016/s0140-6736(05)66658-5
68. Shopland DR (1995) Tobacco use and its contribution to early cancer mortality with a special emphasis on cigarette smoking. Environ Health Perspect 103(Suppl 8):131–142. https://doi.org/10.1289/ehp.95103s8131
69. Chaturvedi AK, Engels EA, Pfeiffer RM, Hernandez BY, Xiao W, Kim E et al (2011) Human papillomavirus and rising oropharyngeal cancer incidence in the United States. J Clin Oncol 29(32):4294–4301. https://doi.org/10.1200/jco.2011.36.4596
70. National Center for Health Statistics (2016) Health, United States, 2015: with special feature on racial and ethnic health disparities, Report No. 2016-1232. National Center for Health Statistics, Hyattsville
71. Grafton-Clarke C, Chen KW, Wilcock J (2019) Diagnosis and referral delays in primary care for oral squamous cell cancer: a systematic review. Br J Gen Pract 69(679):e112–e126. https://doi.org/10.3399/bjgp18X700205
72. Wan A, Savage NW (2010) Biopsy and diagnostic histopathology in dental practice in Brisbane: usage patterns and perceptions of usefulness. Aust Dent J 55(2):162–169. https://doi.org/10.1111/j.1834-7819.2010.01210.x
73. Llewellyn CD, Johnson NW, Warnakulasuriya KA (2001) Risk factors for squamous cell carcinoma of the oral cavity in young people – a comprehensive literature review. Oral Oncol 37(5):401–418. https://doi.org/10.1016/s1368-8375(00)00135-4
74. O'Connor JP, Rose CJ, Waterton JC, Carano RA, Parker GJ, Jackson A (2015) Imaging intratumor heterogeneity: role in therapy response, resistance, and clinical outcome. Clin Cancer Res 21(2):249–257. https://doi.org/10.1158/1078-0432.ccr-14-0990
75. Farah CS, Dost F, Do L (2019) Usefulness of optical fluorescence imaging in identification and triaging of oral potentially malignant disorders: a study of VELscope in the LESIONS programme. J Oral Pathol Med 48(7):581–587. https://doi.org/10.1111/jop.12896
76. Uthoff RD, Song B, Sunny S, Patrick S, Suresh A, Kolur T et al (2018) Point-of-care, smartphone-based, dual-modality, dual-view, oral cancer screening device with neural network classification for low-resource communities. PLoS One 13(12):e0207493. https://doi.org/10.1371/journal.pone.0207493
77. Heidari AE, Pham TT, Ifegwu I, Burwell R, Armstrong WB, Tjoson T et al (2020) The use of optical coherence tomography and convolutional neural networks to distinguish normal and abnormal oral mucosa. J Biophotonics 13(3):e201900221. https://doi.org/10.1002/jbio.201900221
78. Friedman-Kien AE (1981) Disseminated Kaposi's sarcoma syndrome in young homosexual men. J Am Acad Dermatol 5(4):468–471. https://doi.org/10.1016/s0190-9622(81)80010-2
79. Pakfetrat A, Falaki F, Delavarian Z, Dalirsani Z, Sanatkhani M, Zabihi Marani M (2015) Oral manifestations of human immunodeficiency virus-infected patients. Iran J Otorhinolaryngol 27(78):43–54
80. Lancet T (2017) The global HIV/AIDS epidemic-progress and challenges. Lancet 390(10092):333. https://doi.org/10.1016/S0140-6736(17)31920-7
81. HIV in the United Arab Emirates. The Borgen Project. 2019 Dec 18. https://borgenproject.org/hiv-in-the-united-arab-emirates/
82. Indrastiti RK, Wardhany II, Soegyanto AI (2020) Oral manifestations of HIV: can they be an indicator of disease severity? (A systematic review). Oral Dis 26(Suppl 1):133–136. https://doi.org/10.1111/odi.13394
83. Ottria L, Lauritano D, Oberti L, Candotto V, Cura F, Tagliabue A, Tettamanti L (2018) Prevalence of HIV-related oral manifestations and their association with HAART and CD4+ T cell count: a review. J Biol Regul Homeost Agents 32(2 Suppl. 1):51–59
84. Ahlström MG, Ronit A, Omland LH, Vedel S, Obel N (2019) Algorithmic prediction of HIV status using nation-wide electronic registry data. EClinicalMedicine 17:100203. https://doi.org/10.1016/j.eclinm.2019.10.016

85. Krakower DS, Gruber S, Hsu K, Menchaca JT, Maro JC, Kruskal BA et al (2019) Development and validation of an automated HIV prediction algorithm to identify candidates for pre-exposure prophylaxis: a modelling study. Lancet HIV 6(10):e696–e704. https://doi.org/10.1016/s2352-3018(19)30139-0
86. Marcus JL, Hurley LB, Krakower DS, Alexeeff S, Silverberg MJ, Volk JE (2019) Use of electronic health record data and machine learning to identify candidates for HIV pre-exposure prophylaxis: a modelling study. Lancet HIV 6(10):e688–e695. https://doi.org/10.1016/s2352-3018(19)30137-7
87. Wray TB, Luo X, Ke J, Pérez AE, Carr DJ, Monti PM (2019) Using smartphone survey data and machine learning to identify situational and contextual risk factors for HIV risk behavior among men who have sex with men who are not on PrEP. Prev Sci 20(6):904–913. https://doi.org/10.1007/s11121-019-01019-z
88. Young SD, Yu W, Wang W (2017) Toward automating HIV identification: machine learning for rapid identification of HIV-related social media data. J Acquir Immune Defic Syndr (1999) 74(Suppl 2):S128–S131. https://doi.org/10.1097/QAI.0000000000001240
89. Marcus JL, Sewell WC, Balzer LB, Krakower DS (2020) Artificial intelligence and machine learning for HIV prevention: emerging approaches to ending the epidemic. Curr HIV/AIDS Rep 17(3):171–179. https://doi.org/10.1007/s11904-020-00490-6
90. Eweka O, Agbelusi G, Odukoya O (2012) Prevalence of oral lesions and the effects of HAART in adult HIV patients attending a tertiary hospital in Lagos, Nigeria. Open J Stomatol 2:200–205. https://doi.org/10.4236/ojst.2012.23036
91. Petersson EE, Andersson L, Sörensen S (1997) Traumatic oral vs non-oral injuries. Swed Dent J 21(1–2):55–68
92. Akin A, Uysal S, Cehreli ZC (2011) Segmental alveolar process fracture involving primary incisors: treatment and 24-month follow up. Dent Traumatol 27(1):63–66. https://doi.org/10.1111/j.1600-9657.2010.00953.x
93. Top Doctor's United Kingdom. Dental trauma. https://www.topdoctors.co.uk/medical-dictionary/dental-trauma#Treatments
94. Lam R (2016) Epidemiology and outcomes of traumatic dental injuries: a review of the literature. Aust Dent J 61:4–20. https://doi.org/10.1111/adj.12395
95. Da Silva Assunção LR, Ferelle A, Iwakura ML, Cunha RF (2009) Effects on permanent teeth after luxation injuries to the primary predecessors: a study in children assisted at an emergency service. Dent Traumatol 25(2):165–170. https://doi.org/10.1111/j.1600-9657.2008.00759.x
96. Robertson A, Norén JG (2001) Knowledge-based system for structured examination, diagnosis and therapy in treatment of traumatised teeth. Dent Traumatol 17(1):5–9. https://doi.org/10.1034/j.1600-9657.2001.170102.x
97. Ozer S, Yilmaz EI, Bayrak S, Tunc ES (2012) Parental knowledge and attitudes regarding the emergency treatment of avulsed permanent teeth. Eur J Dent 6(4):370–375
98. Bayrak S, Tunc ES, Sari E (2012) Evaluation of elementary school teachers' knowledge and attitudes about immediate emergency management of traumatic dental injuries. Oral Health Prev Dent 10(3):253–258
99. Vidović D, Gorseta K, Bursac D, Glavina D, Skrinjarić T (2014) Taekwondo coaches knowledge about prevention and management of dental trauma. Coll Antropol 38(2):681–684
100. Nasr IH, Papineni McIntosh A, Mustafa S, Cronin A (2013) Professional knowledge of accident and emergency doctors on the management of dental injuries. Community Dent Health 30(4):234–240
101. Djemal S, Singh P (2016) Smartphones and dental trauma: the current availability of apps for managing traumatic dental injuries. Dent Traumatol 32(1):52–57. https://doi.org/10.1111/edt.12217
102. Sajja PS, Akerkar R (2010) Knowledge-based systems for development. Adv Knowl Based Syst Model Appl Res 1:1–11

103. Grischke J, Johannsmeier L, Eich L, Griga L, Haddadin S (2020) Dentronics: towards robotics and artificial intelligence in dentistry. Dental Mater 36(6):765–778. https://doi.org/10.1016/j.dental.2020.03.021
104. Kostiuk MBB (2022 Jan). Trauma assessment. [Updated 2021 Jul 28]. In: StatPearls [Internet]. StatPearls Publishing, Treasure Island. Available from: https://www.ncbi.nlm.nih.gov/books/NBK555913/
105. Kurt Bayrakdar S, Orhan K, Bayrakdar IS, Bilgir E, Ezhov M, Gusarev M, Shumilov E (2021) A deep learning approach for dental implant planning in cone-beam computed tomography images. BMC Med Imaging 21(1):86. https://doi.org/10.1186/s12880-021-00618-z
106. Gampel NE, Punjabi AP (2019 Jan 15) Management of dental trauma. Drug & diseases. Dentistry. https://emedicine.medscape.com/article/1799897-overview
107. Srour ML, Farley E, Mpinga EK (2022) Lao Noma survivors: a case series, 2002–2020. Am J Trop Med Hyg. https://doi.org/10.4269/ajtmh.21-1079
108. Park J, Kim S, Shin SW, Lyu CJ, Kim D (2022) Noma disease (cancrum oris, orofacial gangrene) in an acute myeloid leukemia patient: a case report. J Med Case Rep 16(1):97. https://doi.org/10.1186/s13256-022-03317-7
109. Speiser S, Langridge B, Birkl MM, Kubiena H, Rodgers W (2021) Update on Noma: systematic review on classification, outcomes and follow-up of patients undergoing reconstructive surgery after Noma disease. BMJ Open 11(8):e046303. https://doi.org/10.1136/bmjopen-2020-046303
110. Srour ML et al (2017) Noma: overview of a neglected disease and human rights violation. Am J Trop Med Hyg 96(2):268–274. https://doi.org/10.4269/ajtmh.16-0718
111. Marck KW, de Bruijn HP, Schmid F, Meixner J, van Wijhe M, van Poppelen R (1998) Noma: the Sokoto approach. Eur J Plast Surg 21:277–280
112. Montandon D, Lehmann C, Chami N (1991) The surgical treatment of Noma. Plast Reconstr Surg 87(1):76–86. https://doi.org/10.1097/00006534-199101000-00013
113. Mohammed MI, Cadd B, Peart G, Gibson I (2018) Augmented patient-specific facial prosthesis production using medical imaging modelling and 3D printing technologies for improved patient outcomes. Virtual Phys Prototyping 13(3):164–176. https://doi.org/10.1080/17452759.2018.1446122
114. Jazayeri HE, Kang S, Masri RM, Kuhn L, Fahimipour F, Vanevenhoven R et al (2018) Advancements in craniofacial prosthesis fabrication: a narrative review of holistic treatment. J Adv Prosthodont 10(6):430–439. https://doi.org/10.4047/jap.2018.10.6.430
115. Mine Y, Suzuki S, Eguchi T, Murayama T (2020) Applying deep artificial neural network approach to maxillofacial prostheses coloration. J Prosthodont Res 64(3):296–300
116. Anthony PM, Kahnberg K-E, Andersson L (2014) Essentials of oral and maxillofacial surgery. Wiley Blackwell, Chichester, pp 297–315
117. Kruppa K, Kruger E, Vorster C, der Linde JV (2021) Cleft lip and/or palate and associated risks in lower-middle-income countries: a systematic review. Cleft Palate Craniofac J. https://doi.org/10.1177/10556656211018952
118. Boyles AL, DeRoo LA, Lie RT, Taylor JA, Jugessur A, Murray JC, Wilcox AJ (2010) Maternal alcohol consumption, alcohol metabolism genes, and the risk of oral clefts: a population-based case-control study in Norway, 1996–2001. Am J Epidemiol 172(8):924–931. https://doi.org/10.1093/aje/kwq226
119. Beaty TH, Ruczinski I, Murray JC, Marazita ML, Munger RG, Hetmanski JB et al (2011) Evidence for gene-environment interaction in a genome wide study of nonsyndromic cleft palate. Genet Epidemiol 35(6):469–478. https://doi.org/10.1002/gepi.20595
120. Wu T, Liang KY, Hetmanski JB, Ruczinski I, Fallin MD, Ingersoll RG et al (2010) Evidence of gene-environment interaction for the IRF6 gene and maternal multivitamin supplementation in controlling the risk of cleft lip with/without cleft palate. Hum Genet 128(4):401–410. https://doi.org/10.1007/s00439-010-0863-y
121. Barnes S. Teachme anatomy. Development of the face and palate. https://teachmeanatomy.info/the-basics/embryology/head-neck/face-palate/

122. Nyberg DA, Hegge FN, Kramer D, Mahony BS, Kropp RJ (1993 June) Premaxillary protrusion: a sonographic clue to bilateral cleft lip and palate. J Ultrasound Med 12(6):331–335. https://doi.org/10.7863/jum.1993.12.6.331. PMID: 8515530
123. Young JI, Slifer S, Hecht JT, Blanton SH (2021) DNA methylation variation is identified in monozygotic twins discordant for non-syndromic cleft lip and palate. Front Cell Dev Biol 9:656865. https://doi.org/10.3389/fcell.2021.656865
124. Agarwal S, Hallac RR, Mishra R, Li C, Daescu O, Kane AA (2018) Image based detection of craniofacial abnormalities using feature extraction by classical convolutional neural network. 2018 IEEE 8th international conference on computational advances in bio and medical sciences (ICCABS), pp 1–6
125. Alam MK, Alfawzan AA (2020) Dental characteristics of different types of cleft and non-cleft individuals. Front Cell Dev Biol 8. https://doi.org/10.3389/fcell.2020.00789
126. Alam MK, Alfawzan AA (2020) Evaluation of Sella Turcica bridging and morphology in different types of cleft patients. Front Cell Dev Biol 8. https://doi.org/10.3389/fcell.2020.00656
127. Li Y, Cheng J, Mei H, Ma H, Chen Z, Li Y (2019) CLPNet: cleft lip and palate surgery support with deep learning. Annu Int Conf IEEE Eng Med Biol Soc 2019:3666–3672. https://doi.org/10.1109/embc.2019.8857799
128. Lin G, Kim PJ, Baek SH, Kim HG, Kim SW, Chung JH (2021) Early prediction of the need for orthognathic surgery in patients with repaired unilateral cleft lip and palate using machine learning and longitudinal lateral cephalometric analysis data. J Craniofac Surg 32(2):616–620. https://doi.org/10.1097/scs.0000000000006943
129. Park HM, Kim PJ, Kim HG, Kim S, Baek SH (2015) Prediction of the need for orthognathic surgery in patients with cleft lip and/or palate. J Craniofac Surg 26(4):1159–1162. https://doi.org/10.1097/scs.0000000000001605
130. Schiebl J, Bauer FX, Grill F, Loeffelbein DJ (2020) RapidNAM: algorithm for the semi-automated generation of nasoalveolar molding device designs for the presurgical treatment of bilateral cleft lip and palate. IEEE Trans Biomed Eng 67(5):1263–1271. https://doi.org/10.1109/tbme.2019.2934907
131. Pocket dentistry. Chapter 29: Cleft lip and palate. https://pocketdentistry.com/cleft-lip-and-palate-7/
132. Gaddey HL (2017 Nov–Dec) Oral manifestations of systemic disease. Gen Dent 65(6):23–29. PMID: 29099362
133. Cheraskin E (1958) Oral manifestations of systemic diseases. J Natl Med Assoc 50(4):241
134. Bhalla N, Nudell Y, Thakkar J, Dym H (2020) Oral manifestation of systemic diseases. Dent Clin 64(1):191–207
135. Mavragani CP, Moutsopoulos HM (2014) Sjögren syndrome. CMAJ 186(15):E579–E586
136. Fox RI, Stern M, Michelson P (2000) Update in Sjögren syndrome. Curr Opin Rheumatol 12(5):391–398
137. Porter S, Mercadante V, Fedele S (2017) Oral manifestations of systemic disease. Br Dent J 223(9):683–691
138. Batistella EÂ, Sabino da Silva R, Rivero ERC, Silva CAB (2021) Prevalence of oral mucosal lesions in patients with pemphigus vulgaris: a systematic review and meta-analysis. J Oral Pathol Med 50(8):750–757
139. Kuriachan D, Suresh R, Janardhanan M, Savithri V (2015) Oral lesions: the clue to diagnosis of pemphigus vulgaris. Case Rep Dent 2015:593940
140. Macena M, Praxedes D, De Oliveira AD, Paula D, Barros M, Júnior AS et al (2022) Prevalence of iron deficiency anemia in Brazilian women of childbearing age: a systematic review with meta-analysis. PeerJ 10:e12959
141. Kaur L, Puri M, Saraswathy KN, Trivedi SS, Sachdeva MP (2018) Recurrent pregnancy losses vis-à-vis anemia and vitamin (folate/B12) imbalance. Int J Health Gov 23:281
142. Halim N, Kalkur C, Padmashree S, Rangare AL (2018) Diagnosis of iron deficiency anemia through oral manifestation – a case report. J Online J Case Stud 7(5):5–7
143. DeLoughery TG (2017) Iron deficiency anemia. Med Clin 101(2):319–332

144. Toh B-H, van Driel IR, Gleeson PA (1997) Pernicious anemia. N Engl J Med 337(20):1441–1448
145. Anitha N, Appadurai P, Anitha N (2020) Anemia and it's oral manifestation. Eur J Mol Clin Med 7(8):1715–1719
146. Döhner H, Weisdorf DJ, Bloomfield CD (2015) Acute myeloid leukemia. N Engl J Med 373(12):1136–1152
147. Francisconi CF, Caldas RJ, Oliveira Martins LJ, Fischer Rubira CM, da Silva Santos PS (2016) Leukemic oral manifestations and their management. Asian Pac J Cancer Prev 17(3):911–915
148. Quispe RA, Aguiar EM, de Oliveira CT, Neves ACX, da Silva Santos PS (2021) Oral manifestations of leukemia as part of early diagnosis. Hematol Transfus Cell Ther 44(3):392–401
149. Egeler RM, D'Angio GJ (1995) Langerhans cell histiocytosis. J Pediatr 127(1):1–11
150. Abdull Gaffar B, Awadhi F (2020) Oral manifestations of Langerhans cell histiocytosis with unusual histomorphologic features. Ann Diagn Pathol 47:151536
151. Madrigal-Martínez-Pereda C, Guerrero-Rodriguez V, Guisado-Moya B, Meniz-Garcia C (2009) Langerhans cell histiocytosis: literature review and descriptive analysis of oral manifestations. Med Oral Patol Oral Cir Bucal 14(5):E222–E228
152. Rohani B (2019) Oral manifestations in patients with diabetes mellitus. World J Diabetes 10(9):485
153. Mauri-Obradors E, Estrugo-Devesa A, Jané-Salas E, Viñas M, López-López J (2017) Oral manifestations of diabetes mellitus. A systematic review. Med Oral Patol Oral Cir Bucal 22(5):e586–e594. https://doi.org/10.4317/medoral.21655
154. de Lima DC, Nakata GC, Balducci I, Almeida JD (2008) Oral manifestations of diabetes mellitus in complete denture wearers. J Prosthet Dent 99(1):60–65
155. Islam SMS, Niessen LW, Seissler J, Ferrari U, Biswas T, Islam A, Lechner A (2015) Diabetes knowledge and glycemic control among patients with type 2 diabetes in Bangladesh. Springerplus 4(1):1–7
156. Dar-Odeh NS, Alsmadi OM, Bakri F, Abu-Hammour Z, Shehabi AA, Al-Omiri MK et al (2010) Predicting recurrent aphthous ulceration using genetic algorithms-optimized neural networks. Adv Appl Bioinform Chem 3:7–13. https://doi.org/10.2147/aabc.s10177
157. Peres MA, Macpherson LM, Weyant RJ, Daly B, Venturelli R, Mathur MR et al (2019) Oral diseases: a global public health challenge. Lancet 394(10194):249–260
158. Jin L, Lamster I, Greenspan J, Pitts N, Scully C, Warnakulasuriya S (2016) Global burden of oral diseases: emerging concepts, management and interplay with systemic health. Oral Dis 22(7):609–619
159. Petersen PE, Bourgeois D, Ogawa H, Estupinan-Day S, Ndiaye C (2005) The global burden of oral diseases and risks to oral health. Bull World Health Organ 83:661–669
160. Petersen PE (2003) The World Oral Health report 2003: continuous improvement of oral health in the 21st century – the approach of the WHO Global Oral Health Programme. Community Dent Oral Epidemiol 31:3–24
161. Stone C (2013) Cleft lip and palate: etiology, epidemiology, preventive and intervention strategies. Anat Physiol 4(03). https://doi.org/10.4172/2161-0940.1000150
162. Dye BA (2017) The global burden of oral disease: Research and public health significance. J Dent Res 96(4):361–363. https://doi.org/10.1177/0022034517693567

Chapter 4
Oral Health in Global Health

4.1 What Is Global Health?

Macfarlane et al. describe global health as being the "worldwide improvement of health, reduction of disparities, and protection against global threats that disregard national borders" [1].

- **Proposed Definition**

Proposed definition for global health is *collaborative transnational research and action for promoting health for all.*

The term *global health* is used rather than global public health to avoid the perception that our endeavors are focused only on classical, and nationally based, public health actions. Global health builds on national public health efforts and institutions. In many countries, public health is equated primarily with population-wide interventions; global health is concerned with all strategies for health improvement, whether population-wide or individually based health-care actions, and across all sectors, not just the health sector [2].

- **Global Health: A High-Income Country Concern?**

Although the burden of preventable disease is in middle- and, especially, low-income countries, most global health centers are in high-income countries. There are several explanations for this anomaly including the following [2]:

- Centers in low- and middle-income countries are engaged in global health issues but under other labels. For example, several centers in low- and middle-income countries have recently been funded by the National Heart, Lung, and Blood Institute to undertake chronic disease prevention activities, though the focus is on national programs of work.
- Global health builds on international health interests stemming from institutions in high-income countries over a century ago.

K. Shaikh et al., *Artificial Intelligence in Dentistry*,
https://doi.org/10.1007/978-3-031-19715-4_4

- Global health may be seen to be divorced from the health needs of low- and middle-income countries which are grappling with a range of pressing and challenging health issues.
- An interest in global health stems from strong national public health institutions which are usually not a feature of low- and middle-income countries.

Whatever the explanation, encouraging and supporting the establishment of global health centers in low- and middle-income countries, and south-south collaborations, are essential if countries with the greatest burden of diseases are to have the best opportunity to respond appropriately. Development agencies, foundations, and national ministries of health could do much more to build public health capacity at the national level. By doing so, they will also strengthen research and policy interests in global health and its evaluation [2].

4.2 Oral Health in Global Health

As we mentioned in the previous chapters, though largely preventable, dental caries and periodontal disease are the two biggest threats to oral health and are among the most common chronic diseases. Dental caries is the most common chronic disease in children: it is about five times as common as asthma and seven times as common as hay fever. The most common cause of tooth loss among adults is untreated periodontal disease. Fifty-three million people live with untreated tooth decay in their permanent teeth. Strikingly, one-quarter of adults aged 65 years and older have lost all of their teeth due to untreated oral disease [3].

Despite these statistics, the majority of the population often take oral health for granted. Unknown to many are the complications associated with untreated dental caries and periodontal disease. If left untreated, they may cause pain, dysfunction, poor appearance, loss of self-esteem, absence from school or work, and difficulty concentrating on daily tasks [3].

The health disparities surrounding access to proper dental care add another layer of complexity. The silent epidemic of oral diseases disproportionately affects disadvantaged communities, especially children, the elderly, and racial/ethnic minority groups. Oral health disparities are exacerbated by the fact that a cavity continues to enlarge and become more complex to repair the longer it remains untreated. Only one in five school-aged children from low- income families receives dental sealants to prevent dental caries [3].

Oral diseases are being the most prevalent diseases globally and have serious health and economic burdens, greatly reducing quality of life for those affected. Oral diseases persist with high prevalence, reflecting widespread social and economic inequalities and inadequate funding for prevention and treatment, particularly in low-income and middle-income countries (LMICs). As with most noncommunicable diseases (NCDs), oral conditions are chronic and strongly socially patterned. Children living in poverty, socially marginalized groups, and older people are the most affected by oral diseases and have poor access to dental care. In many LMICs, oral diseases remain largely untreated because the treatment costs exceed available resources. The personal consequences of chronic untreated oral diseases are often severe and can include unremitting pain, sepsis, reduced quality of life, lost school days, disruption to family life, and decreased work productivity. The costs of treating oral diseases impose large economic burdens to families and health-care systems. All these factors make oral diseases undoubtedly a global public health problem, with particular concern over their rising prevalence in many LMICs linked to wider social, economic, and commercial changes. Oral conditions disproportionally affect impoverished and socially disadvantaged members of society. A strong and consistent social gradient exists between socioeconomic status and the prevalence and severity of oral diseases [4].

However, oral health is rarely seen as a priority in health policy. Oral health and the dental profession have become somewhat isolated and marginalized from mainstream developments in health policy and health-care systems. The current model of dental care delivery and clinical preventive policy does not tackle the global burden of oral diseases. The so-called westernized model of modern dentistry (high technology and treatment focused) is unaffordable and inappropriate in many LMICs. Even in settings with resources, dentistry is not meeting the needs of large segments of the national population and is increasingly focusing on the provision of aesthetic treatments, largely driven by profit motives and consumerism. A radically different approach is needed to tackle the global challenge of oral diseases.

Also, an important first step in combating the two leading causes of poor oral health—dental caries and periodontal disease—is understanding that tooth loss is often the result of disease or injury, rather than an inevitable consequence of aging. Educational programs emphasizing the importance of oral health promotion/disease prevention are also necessary to raise awareness and discourage the lack of concern regarding oral health. Proper oral health is vital to a productive and healthy life [3].

Global health is about reaching beyond borders, disciplines, and cultures to tackle health inequalities but also about preparing the health workforce and health systems to the effects of these threats of global dimension [1]. Within this context, the dental profession has a role in addressing the high prevalence of oral conditions and the inequalities in the distribution of and access to dental care, as well as in preparing the workforce and systems for the impact of future threats that aligns with the goals of global health [5].

4.3 Challenges in Global Oral Health

4.3.1 Oral Health Inequalities

Oral diseases disproportionally affect the poor and socially disadvantaged members of society. There is a very strong and consistent association between socioeconomic status (income, occupation, and educational level) and the prevalence and severity of oral diseases. This association exists from early childhood to older age, and across populations in high-, middle-, and low-income countries [6].

- **Prevention**

The burden of oral diseases and other noncommunicable diseases can be reduced through public health interventions by addressing common risk factors [6].

These include:

- Promoting a well-balanced diet low in free sugars and high in fruit and vegetables, and favoring water as the main drink.
- Stopping use of all forms of tobacco, including chewing of areca nuts.
- Reducing alcohol consumption.
- Encouraging use of protective equipment when doing sports and traveling on bicycles and motorcycles (to reduce the risk of facial injuries).

Adequate exposure to fluoride is an essential factor in the prevention of dental caries.

An optimal level of fluoride can be obtained from different sources such as fluoridated drinking water, salt, milk, and toothpaste. Twice-daily tooth brushing with fluoride-containing toothpaste (1000–1500 ppm) should be encouraged along with flossing.

- **Access to Oral Health Services**

Unequal distribution of oral health professionals and a lack of appropriate health facilities in most countries mean that access to primary oral health services is often low. Moreover, even in high-income settings, dental treatment is costly, averaging 5% of total health expenditure and 20% of out-of-pocket health expenditure [6].

- **WHO Response**

The World Health Assembly approved a Resolution on oral health in 2021 at the 74th World Health Assembly. The Resolution recommends a shift from the traditional curative approach toward a preventive approach that includes promotion of oral health within the family, schools, and workplaces and includes timely, comprehensive, and inclusive care within the primary health-care system. The Resolution affirms that oral health should be firmly embedded within the noncommunicable disease agenda and that oral health-care interventions should be included in universal health coverage programs.

The World Health Assembly delegates asked WHO to develop a draft global strategy on tackling oral diseases for consideration by WHO governing bodies in 2022 and by 2023 to translate the global strategy into an action plan for oral health, to develop "best-buy" interventions on oral health, and to explore the inclusion of Noma within the roadmap for neglected tropical diseases 2021–2030. WHO was asked to report back on progress and results until 2031 as part of the consolidated report on noncommunicable diseases.

Much work is needed to bridge the gap between dental research and global health and to get oral health recognized as a population health priority worldwide. The GBD study showed that oral health has not significantly improved over the last three decades throughout the world and remains a major global public health challenge. Clearly, greater efforts and potentially different approaches are needed to promote global oral health. Conventional dental care is characterized by high cost, which may explain why there are 3.5 billion cases of oral conditions worldwide needing attention, why oral health has been neglected, and why dental care has not been included in many health policies. We argue that a global health network for oral health must be harnessed to drive health system reform. The complexity of developing a new cost-effective oral health system, reducing oral health inequities, and integrating oral health into the health agenda requires a broader participation. The WHO may lead the way forward, build coalitions with relevant external actors, and create an inclusive and unifying global oral health network consisting of dental and nondental members with good representation from all parts of society to reach consensus on how to address the problem. The inclusion of multi-institutional dental health organizations, such as the International Association for Dental Research and World Dental Federation, and influential external actors in dentistry, is crucial for this effort to be successful. Such a network can approve and update (if needed) the research strategies proposed here. The GBD should independently monitor progress. The major indicator of success would be a reduction of the number of cases of untreated dental conditions. Oral health policies and dental care should be solidly based on scientific evidence. Health services must continue carrying out and improving the quality of oral health surveys and surveillance to ensure that timely, relevant, and current data are available for compilation and analyses. Oral health researchers must carry out rigorous assessment of evidence for equity in prevention and management of oral conditions. Finally, oral health care needs to move toward more cost-effective approaches to deliver care to all [7].

4.4 Oral Health, General Health, and Quality of Life

The compartmentalization involved in viewing the mouth separately from the rest of the body must cease because oral health affects general health by causing considerable pain and suffering and by changing what people eat, their speech, and their quality of life and well-being. Oral health also has an effect on other chronic diseases. Because of the failure to tackle social and material determinants and incorporate oral health into general health promotion, millions suffer intractable toothache and poor quality of life and end up with few teeth [8].

Health policies should be reoriented to incorporate oral health using sociodental approaches to assessing needs and the common risk factor approach for health promotion. The determinants of oral diseases are known—they are the risk factors common to a number of chronic diseases: diet and dirt (hygiene), smoking, alcohol, risky behaviors causing injuries, and stress—and effective public health methods are available to prevent oral diseases.

In some countries, oral diseases are the fourth most expensive diseases to treat. Treating caries, estimated at US$ 3513 per 1000 children, would exceed the total health budget for children of most low-income countries. The situation for adults in developing countries is worse, as they suffer from the accumulation of untreated oral diseases. There are few efficient dental care systems to cope with their problems, and where there are, the cost is beyond most people's means. Millions with untreated caries have cavities and suppuration, yet planners continue to overlook oral diseases, despite their significant impact on cost and quality of life. This oversight will lead to more decay and expensive, ineffective clinical interventions [8].

Contemporary concepts of health suggest that oral health should be defined in general physical, psychological, and social well-being terms in relation to oral status. Cohen and Jago consider the greatest contribution of dentistry is to improve quality of life. Disruptions in physical, psychological, and social functioning are therefore important in assessing oral health. Traditional measures use mainly clinical indices, though there are alternatives using measures of oral health-related quality of life in sociodental approaches to assessing need [8].

Chronic diseases such as obesity, diabetes, and caries are increasing in developing countries, with the implication that quality of life related to oral health, as well as general quality of life, may deteriorate. Because oral and other chronic diseases have determinants in common, more emphasis should be on the common risk factor approach. The key concept underlying future oral health strategies is integration with this approach, a major benefit being the focus on improving health conditions in general for the whole population and for groups at high risk, thereby reducing social inequities.

By integrating oral health into strategies for promoting general health and by assessing oral needs in sociodental ways, health planners can greatly enhance both general and oral health [8].

4.5 Ending the Neglect of Global Oral Health: Time for Radical Action

Oral diseases are a major global public health problem affecting over 3.5 billion people. However, dentistry has so far been unable to tackle this problem. A fundamentally different approach is now needed. The urgent need for system reform is ineludible. In high-income countries, the current treatment-dominated, increasingly high-technology, interventionist, and specialized approach is not tackling the underlying causes of disease and is not addressing inequalities in oral health. In low-income and middle-income countries (LMICs), the limitations of so- called westernized dentistry are at their most acute; dentistry is often unavailable, unaffordable, and inappropriate for the majority of these populations, but particularly the rural poor. Rather than being isolated and separated from the mainstream healthcare system, dentistry needs to be more integrated, in particular with primary care services. The global drive for universal health coverage provides an ideal opportunity for this integration. Dental care systems should focus more on promoting and maintaining oral health and achieving greater oral health equity. Sugar, alcohol, and tobacco consumption, and their underlying social and commercial determinants, are common risk factors shared with a range of other noncommunicable diseases (NCDs). Coherent and comprehensive regulation and legislation are needed to tackle these shared risk factors. We have to focus on the need to reduce sugar consumption and describe how this can be achieved through the adoption of a range of upstream policies designed to combat the corporate strategies used by the global sugar industry to promote sugar consumption and profits. Combating the commercial determinants of oral diseases and other NCDs should be a major policy priority [9].

4.5.1 Key Recommendations for the New WHO Global Strategy for Oral Health [10]

1. Inclusion and community engagement

Include the diverse voices of people living with oral diseases in policy dialogues, program planning, and evaluations to ensure that needs and views of disadvantaged populations are addressed when designing inclusive, accessible, and affordable oral health-care systems.

2. Place equity and social justice at the core

Addressing oral health inequalities and their root causes must be central in all policies and future initiatives, fully aligned with the goals of primary health care and UHC.

3. Tackle sugars as a major common risk factor

The evidence of the negative impact of sugars on oral health provides an additional framing option to strengthen upstream population-wide measures, together with limiting the risks from other unhealthy foods and commodities as well as countering industry interference with oral health and NCD strategies.

4. Embrace major system reforms

The integration of oral health care within UHC requires essential, cost-effective intervention packages, integrative delivery and financing models, and adaptations in educating oral health professionals.

5. Better data for decision-making

Data-driven and evidence-informed policy decision-making on oral health needs functioning monitoring and evaluation systems that are fully integrated with existing health monitoring and surveillance approaches.

6. Close financing gaps

Oral health-care financing needs to be addressed as part of the overall NCD financing agenda, with special focus on increased public investments in low-income and middle-income countries, combined with reallocation of spending toward cost-effective best-buy interventions.

UHC = universal health coverage, NCD = noncommunicable disease [10].

References

1. Macfarlane SB, Jacobs M, Kaaya EE (2008) In the name of global health: trends in academic institutions. J Public Health Policy 29:383–401
2. Beaglehole R, Bonita R (2010) What is global health? Glob Health Action 3. https://doi.org/10.3402/gha.v3i0.5142
3. Benjamin RM (2010) Oral health: the silent epidemic. Public Health Rep (Washington, DC: 1974) 125(2):158–159. https://doi.org/10.1177/003335491012500202
4. Peres MA, Macpherson LMD, Weyant RJ, Daly B, Venturelli R, Mathur MR, Listl S, Celeste RK, Guarnizo-Herreño CC, Kearns C, Benzian H, Allison P, Watt RG (2019 July 20) Oral diseases: a global public health challenge. Lancet 394(10194):249–260. https://doi.org/10.1016/S0140-6736(19)31146-8. Erratum in: Lancet 2019 Sept 21;394(10203):1010. PMID: 31327369
5. Hugo FN et al (2021) Role of dentistry in global health: challenges and research priorities. J Dent Res 100(7):681–685. https://doi.org/10.1177/0022034521992011
6. WHO News Room/Facts sheet/Oral health. https://www.who.int/news-room/fact-sheets/detail/oral-health
7. Hugo FN, Kassebaum NJ, Marcenes W, Bernabé E (2021) Role of dentistry in global health: challenges and research priorities. J Dent Res 100(7):681–685. https://doi.org/10.1177/0022034521992011
8. Sheiham A. Oral health, general health and quality of life. Posted August 8, 2013 by gilejoyo in health. Tagged: general health, life, oral health. https://gilejoyongfun.wordpress.com/2013/08/08/oral-health-general-health-and-quality-of-life/
9. Watt RG, Daly B, Allison P, Macpherson LMD, Venturelli R, Listl S, Weyant RJ, Mathur MR, Guarnizo-Herreño CC, Celeste RK, Peres MA, Kearns C, Benzian H (2019 July 20) Ending the neglect of global oral health: time for radical action. Lancet 394(10194):261–272. https://doi.org/10.1016/S0140-6736(19)31133-X. PMID: 31327370
10. Benzian H, Guarnizo-Herreño CC, Kearns C, Muriithi MW, Watt RG (2021) The WHO global strategy for oral health: an opportunity for bold action. Lancet 398(10296):192–194., issn 0140-6736,. https://doi.org/10.1016/S0140-6736(21)01404-5

Chapter 5
Advancements in Dentistry

Digital technologies are now integral to daily life, and the world's population has never been more interconnected. Innovation, particularly in the digital sphere, is happening at unprecedented scale. Even so, its application to improve the health of populations remains largely untapped, and there is immense scope for use of digital health solutions.

WHO is harnessing the power of digital technologies and health innovation to accelerate global attainment of health and the well-being. The WHO Global Strategy on Digital Health, adopted in 2020 by the World Health Assembly, presents a roadmap to link the latest developments in innovation and digital health and put these tools to action in order to improve health outcomes.

Part of WHO's strategic vision is for digital health to be supportive of equitable and universal access to quality health services. Digital health can help make health systems more efficient and sustainable, enabling them to deliver good quality, affordable, and equitable care.

These high ideals are challenging to attain, especially for low- and middle-income countries. The purpose of WHO's Global Strategy on Digital Health is to support countries in strengthening their health systems through the application of digital health technologies and achieve the vision of health for all. The strategy is designed to be fit for purpose and for use by all Member States, including those with limited access to digital technologies, goods, and services [1].

5.1 Importance of Technological Advancements in Dentistry

People are still apprehensive to go to the dentist in spite of the fact that everyone knows how crucial oral health is and how strongly it is connected to our overall health. But an armada of new technologies from virtual reality through artificial intelligence (AI) to CRISPR will revolutionize dentistry and our whole attitude

K. Shaikh et al., *Artificial Intelligence in Dentistry*,
https://doi.org/10.1007/978-3-031-19715-4_5

toward oral health in the future. The quest for advancements in dentistry is never ending, and it is important to embrace new technologies and be educated on the associated risks and benefits when used in dentistry. The realization that new and emerging technological innovations may provide alternative treatments to patients while enhancing workflow, increasing production, and improving the quality of care is on the horizon. Like any other health-care sector, dentistry also has entirely transformed due to the establishment of computer-based advanced technologies, new preventive disease measures, and improved diagnostic techniques in the last few years. Digitalization, cloud technology, and new generations of smartphones and other devices with integrated apps help patients track their diseases continuously. Activity trackers, smart watches, glucose monitors, and other wearable biosensor technology have become a part of our lives [2].

5.2 Technologies That Shape the Future of Dentistry

- **Artificial Intelligence**

Applications of AI are becoming a reality that is run-of-the-mill in all areas of modern human life with the exponential rise in health data and the maturing of health-care AI. Dentistry is entering a new stage of its digitization. Such smart algorithms can be integrated within the health-care system to analyze health data, research findings, and treatment techniques to offer diagnostic and therapeutic recommendations for individual patients. Currently, the use of AI is rapidly advancing beyond text-based, image-based dental practice.

Dentists employ software to get insights in clinical decision-making. Also, patient care is becoming more mobile-oriented, and AI-based devices are instrumental in letting the patients oversee their health while easily sharing this data with their dental practitioners. On top of churning health data, AI-based algorithms can help specialists better tend to dental conditions. Researchers in 2019 developed a machine learning method to accurately quantify immune cells in the vicinity of oral cancer cells. This gives better insights into the spread of and resistance to cancer, thereby helping in determining chances of survival. Others are using neural networks to better detect dental decay and periodontal disease from radiographs. Such approaches can become standard practice in the near future. AI applications in health care are boundless [2].

- **Smart Toothbrush**

Smart toothbrushes come embedded with a plethora of technologies such as cameras, pressure sensors, and much more to track the brushing activity and replicate an oral examination procedure during the routine brushing procedure. The dentist can thereby examine the individual's teeth from the camera's data during the brushing activity. Additionally, pressure sensors attached can be utilized to determine if the brushing process is carried out correctly.

All the data can be shared with the dentist in real time, thus increasing the preventive care process.

The smart brush would even take intraoral images, which are then sent over to the server. Artificial intelligence algorithms would analyze these images and scan them for signs of cracks, caries, or any other abnormalities which require a specialist's attention. If the preliminary scans show anything of concern, both the patient and the clinician would be notified via mobile apps, and the suggestion to make an appointment at the dental clinic would be made to the patient [2, 3].

- **Augmented Reality**

Augmentation reality technology offers virtual information in addition to that of the real environment and thus opens new possibilities in various fields. Augmentation reality technology is also widely used in medical education and training. In dentistry, oral and maxillofacial surgery is the primary area of use, where dental implant placement and orthognathic surgery are the most frequent applications. Recent technological advancements are enabling new applications of restorative dentistry, orthodontics, and endodontics.

AR can be paired with a mannequin on which students can perform procedures while receiving immediate feedback as their movements are tracked. This helps them identify faster where they should improve and develop their skills in the process. It can also be used in dental reconstructive and aesthetic procedures in order to help patients know what they will look like after the treatment. Such AR apps use their phone or tablet's camera to overlay virtual depictions of the improved set of teeth prior to the procedure. This allows patients and dentists to configure features of their teeth such as height and spacing to their liking before they even enter the surgery room [2].

- **Virtual Reality**

Not to be confused with AR, virtual reality (VR) completely closes off the outside world with a dedicated headset and immerses the user in a virtual environment. By slipping such a headset on their head, students and aspiring dental surgeons can be transported to the OR from their couch, while patients can visualize a calming landscape while seated at the dreaded dentist's chair to improve their experience.

Today, only a few students can peek over the shoulder of the surgeon during an operation, and it is challenging to learn the tricks of the trade like that. With a virtual reality camera, surgeons can stream operations globally and allow medical students to actually be there in the OR using their VR goggles. Dentistry even outpaced other fields of medicine in adopting this method. The technology can further be used to help dentists build on their empathy skills through simulations putting them in the shoes of their patients or in challenging situations.

On the patient side, VR might be the solution to our dentist's office anxiety as VR can be used as an effective distraction tool in dentistry. Patients wore goggles which displayed calming natural scenes, and remembered the treatments more positively afterward [2].

As tools of digital technology, augmented reality and virtual reality have been adopted in all disciplines of dentistry and dental education. In particular, virtual articulators have allowed for a full analysis of occlusion with dental models that can simulate all mandibular movements in static and dynamic positions. When combined with additional software, virtual articulators can also enhance education and practice, allow for quicker and more precise individualized diagnoses, and enable discussions of dental treatment planning options with patients during their first appointment [4].

- **Virtual Patients**

Training in medicine and dentistry has evolved to embed technology. This has led to increased opportunities to practice clinical skills in simulated environments before undertaking procedures on patients and to improved precision of skills involving dexterity and hand coordination. This is particularly important in areas such as dentistry. This technology allows the user to explore and manipulate computer-generated real or artificial 3D multimedia sensory environments in real time and can be used to gain practical skills. In comparison with traditional, non-technological teaching methods, this could result in more economical, engaging, and reliable training [5].

The use of virtual patients in dental education is gaining acceptance as an adjunctive method to live patient interactions for training dental students. Use of virtual patients can provide an excellent method for learning and honing patient interviewing skills, medical history taking, recordkeeping, and patient treatment planning. Through the use of virtual patient interactive audio/video elements, the student can experience interaction with his or her virtual patients during a more realistic simulation encounter [6].

- **Teledentistry**

Going to hospitals can be cumbersome for patients with special needs or elderly in nursing homes. Another issue is distance: people living in rural areas rarely get access to a dentist, and almost never have the possibility of choice. This can change significantly with the spread of teledentistry.

Teledentistry services provide easier access to oral and dental care, are significantly cheaper for patients, shift toward more reasonable prevention practices, and allow patients to consult otherwise unavailable medical professionals. It also offers an all-in-one teledentistry platform enabling patients to capture images, send relevant information to a dentist remotely, and do a live consult. The dentist might start a video chat with the patient and the caregiver so that the medical professional can see and talk to the patient, build rapport, help connect them, and bring them into the office (if necessary) [2].

The field of dentistry has seen extensive technologic innovations in recent years. Advances have been made in the use of computers, telecommunication technology, digital diagnostic imaging services, devices, and software for analysis and follow-up. Using advanced information technology, the science of dentistry, today, has crossed much longer distances than it was ever able to. New information technology not only has improved the quality of management of dental patients but also has made possible their partial or complete management at distances of thousands of kilometers away from health-care centers or qualified dentists. The entire process of networking, sharing digital information, distant consultations, workup, and analysis is dealt with by a segment of the science of telemedicine concerned with dentistry known as "teledentistry" [7].

- **Smart Teeth**

Implantation of advanced chips within the prosthesis or chipping off part of the existing tooth to implant the chip could monitor numerous factors. These implants would help create "smart teeth" that can detect saliva's pH, food intake, the quantity of acidic beverages and food consumed, blood alcohol level, etc. and analyze the data via artificial intelligence and big data analytics to develop patterns and associations. This could result in a rise in preventive dentistry based on individual patients' recommendations [3].

- **Computer-Assisted Design and 3D Printing**

Computer-aided design (CAD) and computer-aided manufacturing (CAM) have become an increasingly popular part of dentistry over the past 25 years. The technology, which is used in both the dental laboratory and the dental office, can be applied to inlays, onlays, veneers, crowns, fixed partial dentures, implant abutments, and even full-mouth reconstruction. CAD/CAM is also being used in orthodontics.

CAD/CAM technology was developed to solve three challenges. The first challenge was to ensure adequate strength of the restoration, especially for posterior teeth. The second challenge was to create restorations with a natural appearance. The third challenge was to make tooth restoration easier, faster, and more accurate. In some cases, CAD/CAM technology provides patients with same-day restorations [8].

- **Intraoral Camera and Scanners**

Intraoral cameras (IOC) are digital imaging tools used by dentists to create images of the teeth and mouth. The cameras are small enough to fit comfortably into the mouth on the tip of an intraoral wand that can be moved over and around the teeth. Intraoral (inside the mouth) cameras take high-resolution images of the teeth and mouth using a small camera. In most cases, after the images are captured, an imaging software (such as computer-aided design or computer-aided manufacturing (CAD/CAM) applications) is used to piece hundreds of images together to create a digital 3D model of the intraoral cavity.

IOC helps in the revelation of the hidden and overlooked defects in teeth and other parts of the cavity. Dental world constitutes of microstructures that have to be recorded in a detailed manner to perform patient education, documentation of records and treatment, illustration of lectures, publication, and web connectivity of complicated cases. Also, the compliance of the patient can be increased by the use of IOCs in diagnosis, treatment planning, goal setting, oral hygiene instructions, and maintenance [9].

- **Regenerative Dentistry**

Regenerative dentistry focuses on the regeneration of soft and hard tissues by incorporating tissue engineering approaches. It has been defined as "an interdisciplinary field that applies the principles of both engineering and life sciences, toward the development of biological substitutes that restore, maintain, or improve tissue function" [10].

The field of regenerative dentistry challenges the preconceived idea of shedding of teeth with age or with damage and have them replaced by prostheses, with developments that can lead to self-healing teeth and biological therapy for damaged teeth.

Regenerative medicine typically aims to promote and improve the healing of tissues and organs of the human body, to restore the physiological architecture and the main functions lost. The combination of several scientific fields, including tissue engineering and cell biology, has led to the development of novel regenerative therapies that claim to obtain a better repairing, regenerating, and replacing of tissues and organs damaged by chronic and acute diseases, or by severe traumatic injuries. In this landscape, the mesenchymal stem cells (MSCs) have been widely reported to self-regenerate and differentiate toward different tissues, under specific conditions and stimuli. Nowadays, MSCs are routinely used in autologous transplantation: the use of specific molecular effectors and biomimetic scaffolds populated with such MSCs has shown promising results both in vitro and in vivo experiments aimed to achieve a time-effective tissue reconstruction and a functional regeneration of complex organs [11].

- **CRISPR**

CRISPR is an acronym that stands for clustered regularly interspaced short palindromic repeats. It is a groundbreaking genome editing method offered by Mother Nature herself, but researchers have discovered its immense potential only recently. It might become the ultimate weapon against cancer or, more controversially, help design babies in the future. And the field of dentistry will also benefit from the technology [2].

It has a mechanism of correcting genome errors and turning on/off genes in cells and organisms. Most importantly, it plays a crucial function in bacterial defense by identifying and destroying deoxyribonucleic acid (DNA) segments during bacteriophage invasions since the CRISPR-associated protein 9 (Cas9) enzyme recognizes and cleaves invasive DNA sequences complementary to CRISPR. Therefore, researchers employ this biological device to manipulate the genes to develop new therapies to combat systemic diseases. Currently, the most significant advance at the laboratory level is the generation of cell and animal models, functional genomic screens, live images of the cell genome, and defective DNA repairs to find the cure for genetic disorders [12].

- **Robotics in Navigational Surgery**

Advancements in technology and computer science have led to an increase in the use of robotics in navigational surgery for multiple medical specialties. Robotic surgery is constantly evolving, and its applications are continuously expanding. Recently, robot-assisted surgery has been used for dental implant placement. In the United States, the first robotic dental surgery system was cleared by the Food and Drug Administration for dental implant procedures in 2017. At the end of 2017, the world's first autonomous dental implant placement system was developed by Zhao and colleagues in China. This so-called intelligent robot has a high degree of autonomy, can automatically adjust during intraoperative procedures, and can execute surgical tasks directly on patients without any apparent control by a surgeon [13].

- **Nanodentistry**

Nanodentistry is defined as the application of nanotechnology to diagnose, treat, and prevent oral and dental disease. These approaches intend to preserve and improve the dental health. Nanotechnology deals with structures in the range of 1–100 nm and focuses on the development of materials with novel properties often not present in nature. As a result, it is considered as a key technology of the twenty-first century and promised to deliver innovative methods to medicine in general and to dentistry in particular. Clinical studies already deal with nanotechnology-based tooth treatments and innovative nanocontainers for local drug delivery for more efficient treatments. Nanotechnology has already started to have a significant impact in dentistry, namely, in periodontology, implantology, prosthetic dentistry, orthodontics, and endodontics. Nanotechnology will offer sophisticated methods for diagnosis, therapy, and prevention, so that a new era in medicine becomes reality, often termed nanomedicine. These tools will also create the field of nanodentistry, which finally results in an interdisciplinary challenge to efficiently educate and train all specialists in dentistry and related materials science [14].

References

1. WHO. Health topics. Digital health. https://www.who.int/health-topics/digital-health#tab=tab_3. Accessed on 23 May 2022
2. The Medical Futurist. The amazing future of dentistry and oral health. https://medicalfuturist.com/the-amazing- future-of-dentistry-and-oral-health/. Accessed on 23 May 2022
3. What Next Global. The internet of teeth: dentistry the smart way. https://www.whatnextglobal.com/post/the- internet-of-teeth-dentistry-the-smart-way. Accessed on 23 May 2022
4. Özdemir G, Albayrak B, Yüzbaşioğlu E, Ölçer Us Y (2021) Virtual articulators, virtual occlusal records and virtual patients in dentistry. J Exp Clin Med 38(S2):129–135. https://doi.org/10.52142/omujecm.38.si.dent.9
5. Wanyonyi K, Sivabalan J. On medicine, using virtual reality to train dental professionals. https://blogs.biomedcentral.com/on-medicine/2021/03/11/virtual-reality-train-dental-professionals-isrctn/. Accessed on 23 May 2022
6. Cederberg RA, Bentley DA, Halpin R, Valenza JA (2012) Use of virtual patients in dental education: a survey of U.S. and Canadian dental schools. J Dent Educ 76:1358–1364. https://doi.org/10.1002/j.0022-0337.2012.76.10.tb05391.x
7. Jampani ND et al (2011) Applications of teledentistry: a literature review and update. J Int Soc Prev Community Dent 1(2):37–44. https://doi.org/10.4103/2231-0762.97695

8. Davidowitz G, Kotick PG. The use of CAD/CAM in dentistry. Dent Clin N Am 2011 July;55(3):559–70, ix. https://doi.org/10.1016/j.cden.2011.02.011. PMID: 21726690
9. Pentapati KC, Siddiq H (2019) Clinical applications of intraoral camera to increase patient compliance – current perspectives. Clin Cosmet Investig Dent 11:267–278. https://doi.org/10.2147/CCIDE.S192847
10. Jamal H, Elhussein M (2020 Nov 10) Integration of regenerative dentistry into the dental undergraduate curriculum. https://doi.org/10.3389/fdmed.2020.596189
11. Tatullo M (2020 Apr 18) The regenerative dentistry: current approaches and future insights. Cumhuriyet Dent J 23. https://doi.org/10.7126/cumudj.705652
12. Chavez-Granados PA et al (2022) CRISPR/Cas gene-editing technology and its advances in dentistry. Biochimie 194:96–107. https://doi.org/10.1016/j.biochi.2021.12.012
13. Wu Y et al (2019) Robotics in dental implantology. Oral Maxillofac Surg Clin North Am 31(3):513–518. https://doi.org/10.1016/j.coms.2019.03.013
14. Hieber S, Müller B (2012 Nov 1) NanoScience and technology. In Nanodentistry, vol 61. https://doi.org/10.1007/978-3-642-24181-9_5. 978-3-642-24180-2

Chapter 6
Artificial Intelligence and Learning Algorithms

6.1 Artificial Intelligence

Artificial intelligence (AI) is a broad field of computer science that focuses on creating intelligent machines that can accomplish tasks that would normally require human intelligence and is a method of programming a computer, robot, or other object to think like a smart human [34]. AI is the study of how the human brain thinks, learns, makes decisions, and works to solve problems. The goal of artificial intelligence is to improve computer functions that are linked to human understanding, such as reasoning, learning, and problem-solving [41], although capable of intelligently executing things without being expressly directed.

The emergence of artificial intelligence, which is increasingly grabbing the attention of researchers all over the world, has highlighted the last decade as a watershed moment in technological advancement. Every field has embraced artificial intelligence with fervor, and dental science is no exception [33]. With the massive increase in patient-documented information and data, sophisticated software to gather and save this data is becoming increasingly important. Artificial intelligence has several uses in dental and medical science, from taking a patient's history to data processing and then extracting information from the data for diagnosis. While artificial intelligence will never be able to take the place of a dental surgeon, it is crucial to be aware of the possibilities for combining this breakthrough in technology in the future to improve dental practice.

The purpose of artificial intelligence is to simplify human effort and assist us in making better judgments. Artificial intelligence has also been called "our Final Invention," a development that will create actionable products and services that will transform how we live our lives.

K. Shaikh et al., *Artificial Intelligence in Dentistry*,
https://doi.org/10.1007/978-3-031-19715-4_6

6.1.1 The Types of Artificial Intelligence

- **Reactive Machines**

Reactive machines are designed to complete only a limited number of specialized duties (they will react the same way to the same stimuli every time) [30]. Deep Blue, IBM's chess-playing supercomputer, which beat international grandmaster Garry Kasparov in the late 1990s, is a famous example of this type [19]. Deep Blue can recognize all of the pieces on a chessboard and understand how they move. It is capable of predicting what moves it and its opponent will make next. It can also determine the best course of action from a variety of options. It has no sense of the past and no recall of what has occurred previously. Deep Blue skips everything before the present moment [19, 30].

These techniques help AI systems perform better in certain games, but they can't be readily adjusted or transferred to other circumstances. These programmed minds have no idea of the outside world, which means they can't operate outside of the duties they're given and are easily deceived. They can't interact with the environment the way we imagine AI systems doing in the future. Instead, these machines will react in the same way each time they come across a similar event.

Reactive machines cannot build memories or use knowledge learned to impact future judgments; they can only respond to current conditions [19, 30]. Because it is a lacks memory, it cannot depend on prior experiences to influence real-time decision-making. It sees the world immediately, only capable of doing a limited number of specialized tasks. However, intentionally reducing a reactive machine's worldview is not a cost-cutting technique; rather, it implies that this form of AI will be more trustworthy and dependable—it will respond consistently to the same stimuli.

- **Limited Memory**

Artificial intelligence with limited memory can store previous data and predictions, looking into the past for hints on what may happen next. Artificial intelligence with limited memory is more complicated and has more options than reactive machines [26].

Six steps must be followed when using limited memory.

1. Training data must be created.
2. The machine learning model must be created.
3. The model must be able to make predictions.
4. The model must be able to receive human or environmental feedback.
5. That feedback must be stored as data.
6. These stages must be repeated in a cycle.

Reinforcement learning, long short-term memory (LSTM), and evolutionary generative adversarial networks (E-GAN) are the three models that use the limited memory type.

Virtual voice assistants, chatbots, and self-driving cars use this form of AI [22].

- **Theory of Mind**

Until now, theoretically, the technology and scientific capabilities required to advance artificial intelligence to the next level have not yet been developed. This would imply that AI will be able to grasp how people, animals, and other machines feel and make decisions based on self-reflection and determination and then use that knowledge to make their own judgments. In order to create two-way communication between people and artificial intelligence, computers would need to be able to comprehend and process notions such as "mind," "emotional swings in decision-making," and a slew of other psychological concepts in real time. Sophia, the world-renowned robot, is a famous but yet extremely basic example of this technology. While Sophia cannot recognize or interpret human emotion, she can have basic conversations, has picture recognition, and has the capacity to respond to human interactions with the right facial expression, in addition to having an exceptionally humanlike look[9, 14].

So that theory of mind divides between the AI in the present and AI in the future.

- **Self-Awareness**

The ultimate stage for AI to become self-aware will be to build a theory of mind in artificial intelligence, which will happen sometime in the future. This type of artificial intelligence is conscious on a human level and is aware of its own presence in the environment as well as the presence and emotional condition of others. It would be able to deduce what others may require based on not just what they say to them, but also how they say it [27].

In artificial intelligence, self-awareness requires both human and machine researchers to grasp the concept of consciousness and then discover how to reproduce it so that it can be implemented into machines.

Machines with human-level awareness are included in self-aware AI. This type of AI does not exist right now, but it would be the most sophisticated artificial intelligence ever devised by man.

Self-aware AI has the capacity to think for itself, have wants, and comprehend its feelings, in addition to recognizing and replicating humanlike activities [27]. In essence, self-aware AI is a development and extension of theory of mind AI. Self-aware AI takes it a step further by stating that it can and will have self-guided thoughts and reactions, whereas theory of mind primarily concentrates on the features of understanding and reproduction of human behaviors.

6.1.2 How Artificial Intelligence (AI) Works?

AI systems, in general, function by consuming huge volumes of labeled training data, evaluating the data for correlations and patterns, and then using these patterns to forecast future states. By examining millions of instances, a chatbot given examples of text chats may learn to have lifelike dialogues with humans, and an image recognition program can learn to recognize and describe items in photographs [14, 19].

Learning, thinking, and self-correction are the three basic functions that AI works on. Learning function of AI programming is concerned with gathering data and formulating rules for turning it into useful knowledge. Algorithms are rules that give computer equipment step-by-step instructions for completing a certain task.

Thinking or reasoning is concerned with selecting the best algorithm to achieve a given result. Self-correction function of this element of AI programming aims to fine-tune algorithms on a regular basis to guarantee that they provide the most accurate results feasible. Building an AI system entails reversing human qualities and skills in a computer and leveraging its computational prowess to outperform the talented.

To understand how artificial intelligence works, it is necessary to understand the various subdomains of artificial intelligence and understand how those domains could be applied to the various fields of the industry based on the data we have. Each domain should use an algorithm to process the data and generate output [32].

The common subdomains of AI are:

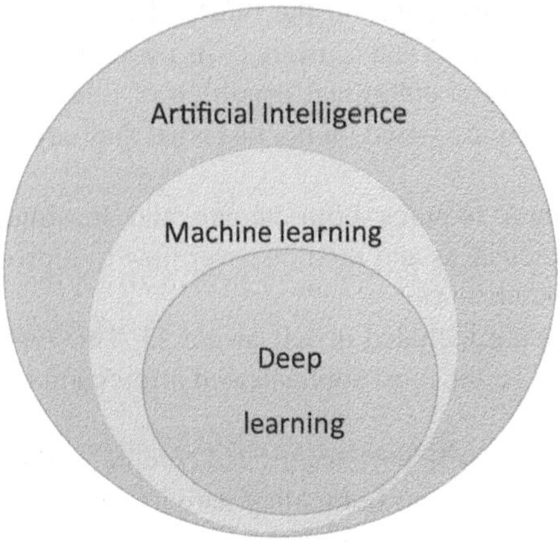

- **Machine Learning (ML)**

It is a popular subdomain of AI; it learns how a machine make a decision based on historical experience and identifies pattern to get the conclusion by evaluating data [13].

- **Deep Learning**

It is a subset of AI, and it is an ML technique. It teaches a machine to process inputs through layers to predict the outcome [32].

The benefits of AIIt is good at detail-oriented work, saves time on data-intensive chores, and consistently produces results, and AI-powered virtual agents are constantly accessible.

6.2 Machine Learning

Machine learning is a subset of artificial intelligence (AI) that encompasses one of AI's key tenets: the potential to learn from experience rather than simply commands. By learning from their output, machine learning algorithms automatically learn and improve, and to generate the desired result, they do not require specific instructions [32]. They learn by observing and comparing their available datasets to examples of the final result, look for patterns in the final output, and attempt to reverse-engineer the facets to generate an output, or in simple words, the process of making machines learn from data to predicting the future output or results and to classify information to try making a right decision, so that machine learning algorithms are trained over instances or examples through which they learn from past experiences and also analyze the historical data.

Machine learning provides data to a computer and uses statistical approaches to help it "learn" how to grow better at a task without being specially programmed for it, obviating the need for algorithms [32]. Machine learning may be used to construct intelligent systems that can make decisions on their own, as well as to improve system efficiency and machine design. These algorithms learn from past data instances through statistical analysis and pattern matching. Then, depending on the learned facts, it tells us the anticipated results. Data is a big part of machine learning algorithms. By training these machine learning algorithms with previous data, we may be able to generate more data [32].

For designing and training machine learning algorithms, AI requires a foundation of specialized hardware and software. Although no one programming language is synonymous with AI, a handful stand out, including Python.

6.2.1 Why Machine Learning?

We can use machine learning to create intelligent systems that can make decisions on their own. Through statistical analysis and pattern matching, these algorithms learn from previous data examples. It then gives us the projected results based on the learned data. The algorithms rely heavily on data. We can produce additional data with the use of past data by training these machine learning algorithms.

Medicine, health care, manufacturing, banking, and a variety of other industries have all been transformed by machine learning. As a result, machine learning has become an important aspect of modern business [12, 48].

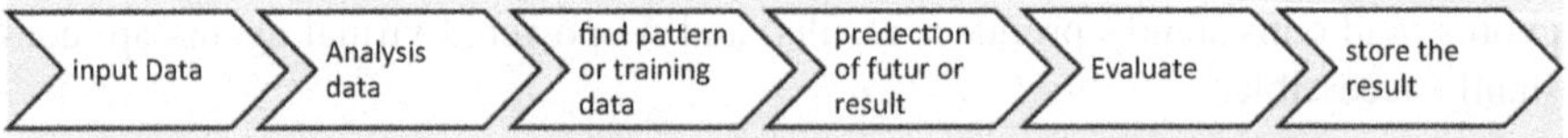

Fig. 6.1 The process of machine learning

Machine learning has introduced another dimension to the way we see information in order to capture the potential of this data, which has been enhanced by the huge rise in processing capacity [44].

6.2.2 How Does Machine Learning Work?

As shown in Fig. 6.1, the first step of machine learning is to input data, which is collected depending on the goals of the project. This step is very important because without data, there is no machine learning, and we have to be sure that the data is complete and correct to avoid any error in the output.

The second step is to analyze the data which involves preparing, cleaning, and manipulating the data. Real-world data are often found unstructured with missing and noisy aspects. Therefore, it has to be cleaned and manipulated to be ready for analysis. This is a crucial step of the machine learning process, and people generally spend most of the time at this step. After data preparation, it needs to be transformed into suitable formats to be aligned with the machine learning platform. Then you divide your data into two sets: training and testing.

In the following stage, the training set is used to train the model.

The third step is to find pattern or train model; the magic happens in this step. The dataset is linked to an algorithm, which develops predictions by utilizing complex mathematical modeling. The fourth step is the prediction of future results. Machine learning algorithms forecast the future based on the patterns seen in the training data. When the ML model receives a new input, it applies its learned patterns to the new data to create future predictions. Various standardized procedures may be used to optimize models based on the end accuracy. After prediction, the result is tested to evaluate ML model performance and also identify bugs and find areas of improvement. We check the model's accuracy. If the results are not satisfactory, you need to improve and retrain your ML model. The last step is to store the result. This result could be used as input in another model or program or can be used in many applications [44].

To make the study of machine learning easy to understand, it is broken out into three main parts.

1. *Decision Process*: Machine learning algorithms are used to create predictions or classifications in general. Your algorithm will provide an estimate of the pattern in the data based on some input data, which can be labeled or unlabeled.

2. *Error Function*: The model's prediction is evaluated using an error function. If there are known instances, an error function may be used to compare the model's accuracy.
3. *Model Optimization Process*: If the model can fit better to the data points in the training set, then weights are adjusted to reduce the discrepancy between the known example and the model estimate. This assessed and optimized procedure will be repeated by the algorithm, which will update weights on its own until a certain level of accuracy is reached.

Machine learning methods employ the same set of characteristics to describe every occurrence in every dataset. The characteristics might be continuous, categorical, or binary [44].

6.2.3 What Factors Should You Consider While Selecting a Machine Learning Model?

If not done on purpose, the process of selecting the correct machine learning model to tackle a problem may be time consuming [39].

Step 1: Align the problem with potential data inputs that should be considered for the solution. This phase needs the assistance of data scientists and specialists with in-depth knowledge of the problem.

Step 2: Gather data, prepare it, and label it as needed. Typically, data scientists lead this process, with assistance from data wranglers.

Step 3: Select the algorithm(s) to be used and evaluate their performance. Data scientists are generally in charge of this stage.

Step 4: Continue to fine-tune the outputs until they are sufficiently accurate. This process is often carried out by data scientists with input from professionals with in-depth knowledge of the topic.

Types of Machine Learning Algorithms Supervised learning.

- Unsupervised learning.
- Reinforcement learning.

6.2.4 Supervised Learning

Supervised learning or supervised learning machine is one of the popular methods used in machine learning; it uses labeled datasets to train algorithms that properly identify data or predict outcomes [8]. As more data is introduced into the model, the weights are adjusted until the model is well fitted. This happens throughout the cross-validation process to verify that the model does not overfit or underfit.

Organizations may use supervised learning to tackle a range of real-world challenges at scale. Neural networks, naive Bayesian (NB) network, linear regression, logistic regression, random forest, support vector machine (SVM), and other approaches are used in supervised learning [8].

Supervised learning uses labeled examples to apply what they've learned in the past to refresh data in order to anticipate future occurrences [28]. The learning algorithm creates an inferred function to generate predictions about the output values based on the examination of a known training dataset. After enough training, the system can offer objectives for any new input. The learning algorithm may also compare its output to the proper, intended output and detect faults, allowing the model to be modified as needed [28]. The input and output are both provided for the supervised learning algorithms and the program looking for connection between it.

The supervised learning algorithm is given a set of inputs and the proper outputs, and it learns by comparing its actual output to the correct outputs in order to detect mistakes. It then makes the necessary changes to the model. Supervised learning employs patterns to predict the values of the label on further unlabeled data using methods like *classification, regression, prediction, and gradient boosting*. The past data predicts expected future events [8, 28] (Fig. 6.2).

6.2.5 *Unsupervised Learning*

Unsupervised learning is used when the information utilized to teach isn't classified or labeled. Unsupervised learning investigates how computers might predict a pattern from unlabeled data to describe a hidden structure. The system doesn't figure

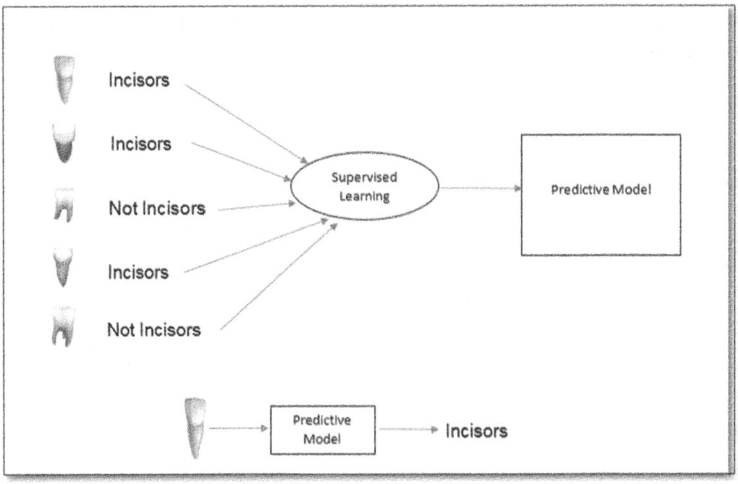

Fig. 6.2 Supervised learning

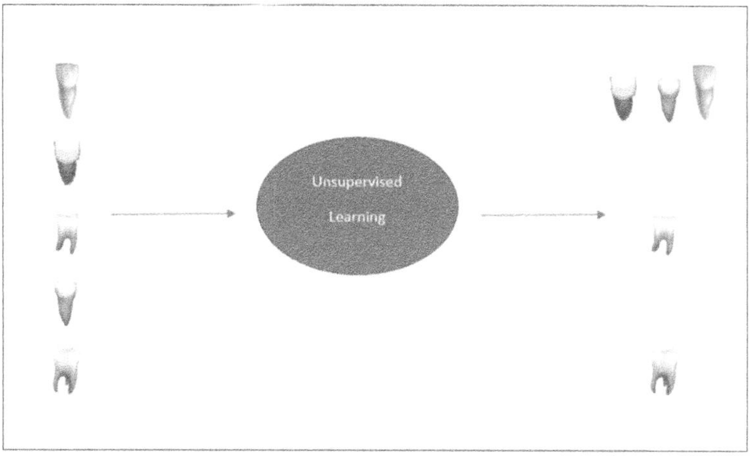

Fig. 6.3 Unsupervised learning

out the proper output, but it examines the data and can predict hidden structures from unlabeled data using datasets [11].

It is used to analyze data that hasn't been labeled previously. The "correct answer" is not given to the system. The algorithm must determine what is being displayed. The idea is to look over the data and see if there is any structure there. On transactional data, unsupervised learning performs effectively. *Self-organizing maps, nearest-neighbor mapping, k-means clustering, and singular value decomposition* are all popular methods used in unsupervised learning [11]. These methods are also employed in the segmentation of text subjects, the recommendation of items, and the detection of data outliers (Fig. 6.3)

6.2.6 Reinforcement Learning

Reinforcement learning is a type of learning that interacts with its surroundings by performing activities and detecting faults or rewards [1, 46]. The most important elements of reinforcement learning are trial and error search and delayed reward. This technology enables machines and software agents to automatically select the best behavior in a given situation in order to improve their efficiency. For the agent to learn which action is better, simple reward feedback is necessary; this is known as the reinforcement signal [1, 46].

Robotics, games, and navigation all employ reinforcement learning. The program uses reinforcement learning to figure out which activities result in the most rewards through trial and error. The agent (the learner or decision-maker), the environment (everything the agent interacts with), and actions are the three main components of this type of learning (what the agent can do). The agent's goal is to select activities that maximize the predicted reward over a set period of time. By following a good policy, the agent will be able to achieve the goal much more quickly [4]. In reinforcement learning, the aim is to learn the optimum policy.

Reinforcement learning guides you through the process of learning a real-world problem by using rewards and penalties as reinforcements. In an ideal world, there is a job or activity that must be taught or done. If the model completes the task, it is rewarded; if it fails, it is penalized. The challenge with reinforcement learning is determining which kind of rewards and punishment are appropriate for the model [45].

6.3 Supervised Learning Algorithms

Supervised learning is a subcategory of machine learning (ML) where training algorithms are given labeled sample inputs with the labels indicating the intended result. Supervised machine learning (SML) looks for algorithms that produce general hypotheses to solve a specific problem and that make predictions about future situations [35].

Supervised learning generates a function that maps inputs to desired outputs. As input data is given into the model, the weights are adjusted until the model is well fitted, which occurs as part of the cross-validation process. Supervised learning assists enterprises in solving a wide range of real-world issues on a large scale, such as categorizing spam in a distinct folder from your email [35]. Labeling an email as spam or not spam is a famous example of this. A multiclass challenge occurs when multiple classes must be learned.

Supervised learning algorithms measure accuracy through the loss function, adjusting until the error has been sufficiently minimized to solve a problem with label data to get the output. The learning algorithm can also compare its output with the correct, intended output and find errors in order to modify the model accordingly. The aim is to make sense of data within the context of a specific question. In other words, supervised learning focuses on creating a compact model of the distribution of class labels based on predictive characteristics [35].

The supervised learning process or how to solve a real-world problem is shown in Fig. 6.4.

After defining the problem, the first step is to collect data, and it's always better to have too much data than too little.

To collect a good and useful data, some questions should be answered to suggest which fields (attributes, features) are the most informative:

1. Do we have a label data?
2. What objectives do I hope to achieve with the use of SML?
3. Do I need the system to be able to forecast anything or only detect patterns?

The second step is to prepare, process, and clean the data according to what the model needs and according to the expected result.

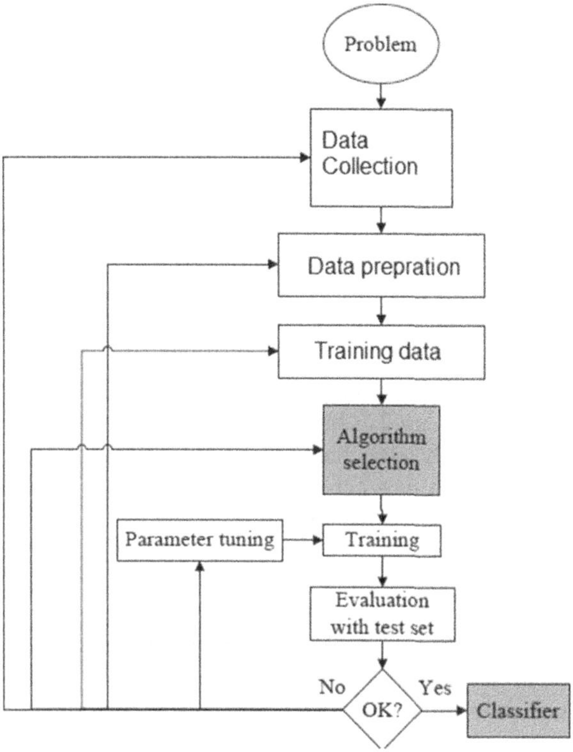

Fig. 6.4 The process of supervised machine learning

After data processing, training data comes which is extremely large label dataset that is used to teach supervised learning and to train a model for prediction or classification of values that are known. The critical step in supervised learning process is to select or choose the specific learning algorithm. The classifier (which maps unlabeled examples to classes) becomes accessible for normal usage once preliminary testing is deemed adequate. Prediction accuracy (the proportion of right predictions divided by the total number of predictions) is frequently used to evaluate the classifier. At least three methods exist for calculating the accuracy of a classifier. One method is to divide the training set in half and use two-thirds for training and the other third for performance estimation. Cross-validation is a technique in which the training set is partitioned into mutually exclusive and equal-sized subsets, and the classifier is trained on the union of all the other subsets for each subset [35]. As a result, the average of each subset's error rate is used to estimate the classifier's error rate. Cross-validation with a single exception is known as leave-one-out validation. There is just one case in each of the test subsets. Of course, this method of validation is more computationally expensive, but it is beneficial when the most exact estimate of a classifier's error rate is necessary.

We must return to an earlier step of the supervised ML process if the error rate evaluation is inadequate (as detailed in Fig. 6.1). A number of things must be considered: if important characteristics for the problem aren't being used, a larger training set is required, the problem's dimensionality is too high, the method used is ineffective, or parameter adjustment is required. Another issue could be that the data is unbalanced.

Statistical comparisons of the accuracy of trained classifiers on specific datasets are a frequent way of comparing supervised ML systems. We may sample a number of training sets of size N, run the two learning algorithms on each of them, and then assess the difference in accuracy for each pair of classifiers on a big test set if we have a significant quantity of data. This differences' average is an estimate of the predicted difference in generalization error across all potential training sets of size N, and their variance is an estimate of the classifier's variance in the entire set [8, 28].

The paired t-test is then used as the next step to test the null hypothesis that the mean difference between the classifiers is zero. This test has the potential to generate two sorts of mistakes. A type I error occurs when the test mistakenly rejects the null hypothesis (i.e., it finds a "significant" difference when there is none). The likelihood that the null hypothesis is not rejected when there is a difference is referred to as a type II error. Type I error of the test will be close to the specified significance threshold.

In fact, we frequently have just one dataset of size N, from which all estimations must be produced. Subsampling is used to create different training sets, and the instances that were not sampled for training are utilized for testing. Regrettably, this contradicts the independence assumption, which is required for adequate significance testing. As a result of this, type I errors exceed the significance level. This is troublesome since it is critical for the researcher to be able to limit type I mistakes and understand the likelihood of rejecting the null hypothesis mistakenly. To address this issue, several heuristic variations of the t-test have been devised.

We'd like the test's result to be independent of the precise partitioning that comes from the randomization procedure because it would make it much easier to duplicate published experimental results. However, there is always some sensitivity to the partitioning employed in practice. To determine replicability, we must run the same test on the same data numerous times with various random partitioning —generally ten times—and count how many times the result is the same.

The main types of supervised learning problems are regression where the output is numerical and classification where the output is categorical.

6.3.1 Classification

A classification problem when the output is category such as "yes" or "no," "black" or "white," "danger" or "no danger," and "happy" or "sad" or "angry" so that classification algorithms used for binary classifications and categorizing. Because the aim is to frequently encourage the computer to learn a classification system that was built, supervised learning is popular in classification challenges. Depending on the labeled data that is trained on supervised learning algorithm, the inputs sort into a given number of categories or classes. By looking at multiple input-output examples of the function, the learner must learn a function that translates a vector into one of several classes.

Classification uses an algorithm to accurately assign test data into specific categories. Common classification algorithms are linear classifiers, support vector machines (SVM), decision trees (DT), k-nearest neighbor (kNN), and random forest [35, 38].

6.3.2 Regression

A regression problem is where the model predicts the output as a continuous numerical or real value, such as "dollars" or "weight" and "price." Both input characteristics and output labels are used to train the algorithm. By estimating how one variable influences the other, it aids in the establishment of a link between the variables. It is utilized to figure out how dependent and independent variables interact. It's widely used to produce forecasts, such as for a company's sales revenue. Popular regression techniques include linear regression, logistical regression, and polynomial regression [5].

The most famous algorithms used to solve the two problems in supervised learning are the following:

- **Liner Classifiers**

One of the most popular algorithms used in solving classification problems, linear classification models use linear (hyperplane) decision boundaries to divide input vectors into classes. The purpose of classification in machine learning with linear classifiers is to arrange objects with comparable feature values into groups. A linear classifier achieves this purpose by producing a classification judgment based on the value of the linear combination of characteristics, according to the statement. Because it is the quickest classifier, a linear classifier is frequently employed in cases where classification speed is a concern.

When the number of dimensions is enormous, such as in document classification, where each element is often the number of counts of a word in a document, linear classifiers frequently perform well. The rate of convergence between dataset variables, on the other hand, is determined by the margin. The margin, in a nutshell, measures how linearly separable a dataset is and hence how simple it is to solve a specific classification issue [16].

- **Support Vector Machines (SVMs)**

These are the most modern techniques for supervised machine learning. SVM models are similar to multilayer perceptron neural networks. SVMs are based on the concept of a margin, which is the distance between two data classes on each side of a hyperplane. It has been demonstrated that increasing the margin and therefore providing the greatest feasible space between the separating hyperplane and the instances on either side of it reduces the predicted generalization error [42].

- **Decision Tree**

Decision trees (DT) are classification trees that order instances based on feature values. Each branch in a decision tree indicates a value that the node might adopt, and each node represents a feature in an instance to be categorized. Starting at the root node, instances are categorized and arranged depending on their feature values [15].

A decision tree is a prediction model that translates observations about an object into inferences about the item's target value in decision tree learning, which is used in data mining and machine learning. Classification trees or regression trees are more descriptive names for such tree models. Post-pruning approaches are commonly used in decision tree classifiers to evaluate the performance of decision trees after they have been pruned using a validation set. Any node can be deleted, and the most common class of the training instances is sorted to be assigned to it [15].

The decision tree models may be used with any data that has both numerical and categorical properties. Nonlinear interactions between features and the goal variable are well captured by decision trees. Because decision trees resemble human thought patterns, understanding the data is simple. The advantages of DT are visually intuitive and simple to understand and analyze. It has the ability to operate with both numerical and categorical data. There is no requirement for one-hot encoding, error terms, or any data preparation. The disadvantage is that any change in data causes a big difference in the structure, which needs changing the implementation.

- **Neural Networks**

A neural network is a set of algorithms that attempt to detect underlying relationships in a batch of data using a method that mimics how the human brain works. Neural networks, in this context, refer to systems of neurons that can be organic or artificial in nature [47].

Multiple neural networks (NN) can execute many regression and/or classification tasks at the same time, despite the fact that most networks can only do one at a time. In the great majority of situations, the network will have only one output variable, albeit this may equate to a number of output units in the case of many state classification issues (the post-processing stage takes care of the mapping from output units to output variables). The input and activation functions of the unit, the network design, and the weight of each input link are all important features of the artificial neural network (ANN) [5].

Given that the first two features are constant, the ANN's behavior is determined by the weights' present values. The training net's weights are set to random values at first, and then instances of the training set are regularly exposed to the net. The values for an instance's input are placed on the input units, and the net output is compared to the instance's desired output. The weights in the net are then modified slightly in the direction of bringing the net's output values closer to the intended output values. A network may be taught using a variety of algorithms [5].

The benefits of artificial neural networks are they are easy to comprehend for professionals who do not wish to go into sophisticated machine learning techniques using arithmetic, are simple to comprehend, are able to recognize all possible interactions between predictor variables, and have the capacity to detect complicated nonlinear interactions between independent and dependent variables in a subtle manner and it's simple to include past information into the model [5, 47].

Artificial neural networks have disadvantages also, i.e., they are extremely difficult to reverse-engineer; artificial neural network methods are not probabilistic, which means that converting a continuous value into a probability is challenging; and artificial neural network techniques with several layers are difficult to train and need a lot of parameter adjustment.

Figure 6.5 shows a simple neural network component.

- **Naive Bayesian (NB) Networks**

This is a typical Bayes' theorem-based probabilistic classifier. Depending on the structure of the probability model, the NB classifier can be trained relatively efficiently in a supervised learning context. When there is no reliance between a single characteristic and other features, given the class, it is considered an optimum classifier. It has been shown to be a good classifier in a broad range of areas despite its simplicity.

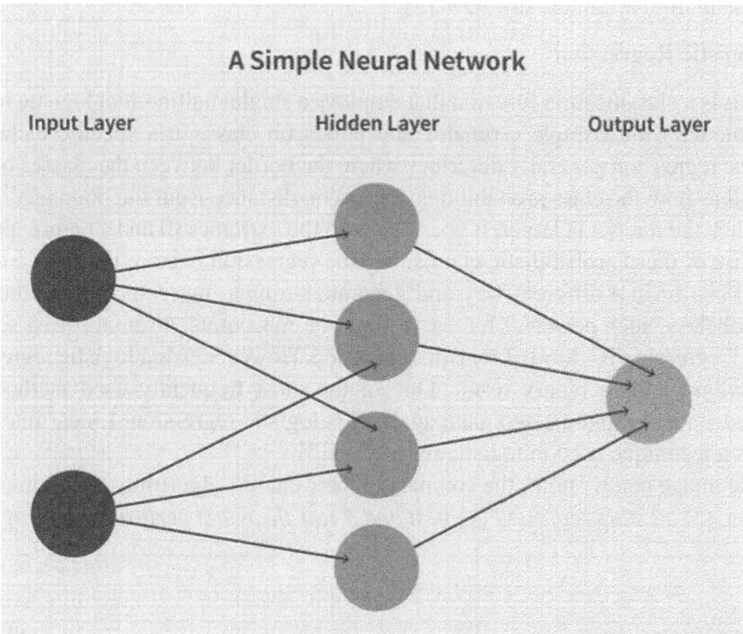

Fig. 6.5 Simple neural network

These are very basic Bayesian networks made up of directed acyclic graphs with just one parent (representing the unseen node) and multiple children (representing observed nodes) with a strong assumption of child node independence in the context of their parent [5].

- **Multilayer Perceptron**

Instead of addressing a non-convex, unconstrained minimization problem as in traditional neural network training, the weights of the network are discovered by solving a quadratic programming problem with linear constraints [40]. Perceptron is also used in other well-known algorithms. The perceptron algorithm is used to learn from a batch of training examples by repeatedly running it over the training set until it finds a prediction vector that is correct across the board. The labels on the test set are then predicted using this prediction rule [40].

- **K-Means**

The k-means method is one of the most basic unsupervised learning techniques for resolving the well-known clustering issue [3]. The approach employs a basic and straightforward method for classifying a given dataset using a predetermined number of clusters (assuming k clusters). When labeled data is not available, the k-means method is used. A general method for converting sloppy guesses into highly precise prediction rules. With enough data and a weak learning algorithm that can consistently find classifiers (rules of thumb) that are at least somewhat better than random, say, accuracy, at 55%, a boosting algorithm may generate a single classifier with extremely high accuracy, say, 95% [3].

- **Logistic Regression**

This is a classification function that employs a single multinomial logistic regression model with a single estimator and builds on class. In a specific technique, logistic regression generally describes where the border between the classes occurs, as well as how the class probabilities depend on distance from the boundary.

When the dataset is larger, it goes closer to the extremes (0 and 1) more quickly. Because of these probabilistic claims, logistic regression is more than just a classifier. It can fit in a different way and generate stronger, more specific predictions. Nevertheless, such powerful forecasts might be inaccurate. Ordinary least squares (OLS) regression is a kind of logistic regression. However, using logistic regression, prediction yields a binary result. One of the most frequently used methods for applied statistics and discrete data analysis is logistic regression. Linear interpolation is a technique used in logistic regression [5].

The image below shows the comparison between the algorithms mentions in this section. *(**** stars represent the best and * star the worst performance)* (Fig. 6.6).

	Decision Trees	Neural Networks	Naïve Bayes	kNN	SVM	Rule-learners
Accuracy in general	**	***	*	**	****	**
Speed of learning with respect to number of attributes and the number of instances	***	*	****	****	*	**
Speed of classification	****	****	****	*	****	****
Tolerance to missing values	***	*	****	*	**	**
Tolerance to irrelevant attributes	***	*	**	**	****	**
Tolerance to redundant attributes	**	**	*	**	***	**
Tolerance to highly interdependent attributes (e.g. parity problems)	**	***	*	*	***	**
Dealing with discrete/binary/continuous attributes	****	***(not discrete)	***(not continuous)	***(not directly discrete)	**(not discrete)	***(not directly continuous)
Tolerance to noise	**	**	***	*	**	*
Dealing with danger of overfitting	**	*	***	***	**	**
Attempts for incremental learning	**	***	****	****	**	*
Explanation ability/transparency of knowledge/classifications	****	*	****	**	*	****
Model parameter handling	***	*	****	***	*	***

Fig. 6.6 Comparing learning algorithms. (**** stars represent the best and * star the worst performance)

6.4 Unsupervised Learning Algorithms

Unsupervised learning is a subcategory of machine learning (ML) where there is input data and no corresponding output variables [6]. It uses algorithms to discover hidden patterns in data without human intervention. It is unlike supervised learning, where there is no correct answer, no label data, an unknown output, and no teacher. This is particularly useful when subject matter experts don't know what to look for in the data and when they are unsure of common properties within a dataset [7].

Unsupervised learning algorithms attempt to mine for rules, recognize patterns, summarize, and aggregate data points in order to derive meaningful insights and better represent the data to consumers using techniques applied to the input data. Unsupervised learning's purpose is to model the data's underlying structure or distribution in order to learn more about it. Algorithms organize data into clusters to represent its structure and make complicated data appear simple and well-organized for examination. It is used for data that hasn't been labeled previously. The "correct answer" is never given to the computer. What is being presented must be determined by the algorithm. The objective is to look at the data and see whether there is any structure there. On transactional data, unsupervised learning excels [6].

The advantages of using unsupervised algorithm are there is no one goal for output and the unlabeled data are more than the labeled data. Unsupervised learning algorithms used k-means, hierarchical agglomerative, and the algorithm based on self-organization map (SOM) neural networks to solve the problem [36].

The main types of unsupervised learning problems are clustering, association, and dimensionality reduction.

6.4.1 Clustering

Cluster analysis is the technique of putting "similar" items together to form "natural" groupings. It is an approach for classifying unlabeled data into groups based on similarities or differences and is the greatest illustration of categorization. Clustering brings together comparable items or data to form distinct clusters and also aids in the detection of dataset biases. Biases are dataset dependencies that connect the occurrence of values in some way. The purpose is to locate homogenous subgroups within the data, with grouping based on the distance between observations [43].

A clustering problem is one in which you wish to uncover the data's inherent groups, such as categorizing clients based on their shopping habits. The general procedure is as follows: given the number of clusters k, an initial partition is created; the clustering solution is then refined repeatedly by transferring documents from one cluster to another. The most prominent partitional method, k-means, and its version, bisecting k-means, have been demonstrated to outperform agglomerative hierarchical algorithms when employed to cluster texts. Clustering algorithms can be categorized into exclusive and overlapping clustering, hierarchical, and probabilistic. The k-means algorithm is generally the most known and used clustering method [31].

- Exclusive and Overlapping Clustering

Exclusive clustering is a type of grouping in which a data point can only be found in one cluster at a time. This type of clustering is often known as "hard" clustering. Exclusive clustering is demonstrated via the k-means clustering technique [31].

K-means clustering is a popular example of an exclusive clustering approach in which data points are assigned to k groups based on the distance from each group's centroid [25]. The data points that are closest to a specific centroid will be grouped together. Smaller groups with greater granularity are indicated by a higher k value, whereas bigger groupings with less granularity are indicated by a lower k value. Market segmentation, document clustering, picture segmentation, and image compression all employ k-means clustering[25].

The method uses a predetermined number of clusters, k, to process a given dataset. The k-means method produces k groups, each with input data partitioned among them.

The k-means algorithm is broken down into the following steps:

1. Enter k for the number of clusters.
2. Pick k data points at random and allocate them to the clusters.

3. Cluster centroids will be determined later.
4. Repeat steps 1–3 until you discover the ideal centroid, after which the numbers will not change.

The k-means clustering ML algorithm has a number of advantages.

- K-means provides tighter clusters than hierarchical clustering in the case of globular clusters.
- For a high number of variables, k-means clustering computes quicker than hierarchical clustering when k is less.

- Hierarchical Clustering

Hierarchical clustering, commonly known as hierarchical cluster analysis (HCA), is an unsupervised clustering technique that may be divided into two types: agglomerative and divisive clustering. Agglomerative clustering is a "bottoms-up" technique to clustering. Its data points are first isolated as independent groups and then blended together repeatedly based on similarity until a single cluster is created [29]. Commonly, different methods are used to measure similarity and to find the distance between two clusters like Ward's linkage, average linkage, complete linkage, and single linkage [29].

- Probabilistic Clustering

A probabilistic model aids density estimation by clustering data points based on their likelihood of belonging to a given distribution. One of the most often used probabilistic clustering algorithms is the Gaussian mixture model (GMM) [10].

Gaussian mixture models are classed as mixture models, which are composed of an unknown number of probability distribution functions. GMMs are most commonly used to figure out which Gaussian or normal probability distribution a particular data point belongs to. We can tell which distribution a particular data point belongs to if we know the mean or variance. However, because these factors are unknown in GMMs, we presume that a latent, or hidden, variable exists to correctly cluster data points. While the expectation-maximization (EM) technique is not needed, it is frequently used to estimate the assignment probability for a given data point to a certain data cluster [10].

6.4.2 Association

It is a form of unsupervised learning technique that uses several rules to discover correlations between variables in a dataset. It's a rule-based approach to discovering correlations between variables in a dataset. These techniques are commonly employed in market basket analysis, helping businesses to better understand the linkages between various items [7]. It is where you want to discover rules that describe large portions of your data, such as people that buy X also tend to buy Y. Businesses may build stronger cross-selling tactics and recommendation engines by understanding their consumers' consumption patterns. The Apriori method is the most extensively used of several algorithms for generating association rules, including Apriori, Eclat, and FP-Growth [7].

- Apriori Algorithms

Market basket analyses popularized Apriori algorithms, resulting in a variety of recommendation engines for music platforms and online stores. They are used to find frequent itemsets, or groups of items, in transactional datasets to determine the chance of consuming a product based on the consumption of another product. This is based on both my own and others' past listening patterns. Apriori methods count itemsets using a hash tree and navigate over the dataset in a breadth-first way [50].

To understand how the Apriori algorithms work, first we must comprehend a few crucial terminologies. The term "itemset" refers to a grouping of objects. The term "n itemset" refers to a collection of n objects. Simply said, it is the collection of items that customers have purchased. Support: It is the proportion of all transactions in which X and Y occur together. Confidence is defined as the degree of assurance that any found rule has. It's the percentage of transactions that have both X and Y out of all transactions that have both X and Y. Lift: It is a measurement of how X and Y are connected rather than how they happen to happen at the same time. It calculates how many times more frequently X and Y occur together than would be predicted if they were statistically independent. When analyzing the algorithm's outcomes, we'll pay special attention to this metric [17].

The rule's minimal number of elements is called minlen. The maximum number of elements in the rule is called maxlen. The term "target" refers to the sort of relationship that was discovered. Frequent itemsets generation: Using specified support and minimum and maximum item values, get the most frequent itemsets from the data. This stage entails producing all of the rules from frequently used itemsets. Controlling support, confidence, or lift can help us limit the number of rules created. LHS > RHS: The terms "left-hand side" and "right-hand side" are commonly used to describe how frequently item A and item B appear together. If we want to know how often consumers visit store A after visiting store B, LHS would be Store A, while RHS would be Store B. Similarly, if we want to know which stores customers normally go to before going to store A, we may put Store A on the RHS and the other businesses on the LHS [17].

6.4.3 Dimensionality Reduction

It's a learning strategy that's employed when a dataset's number of features (or dimensions) is too large [20]. It keeps the data integrity while reducing the amount of data inputs to a tolerable size. When autoencoders remove noise from visual data to enhance picture quality, this approach is frequently utilized in the preprocessing data stage, with the purpose of identifying patterns in the data's characteristics.

Dimensionality reduction is frequently used as a preprocessing strategy before supervised learning to make data easier to see [20].

While more data typically gives more accurate findings, it can also have an influence on the performance of machine learning algorithms (e.g., overfitting) and make dataset visualization more challenging. When the number of characteristics, or dimensions, in a dataset is too large, dimensionality reduction is performed. It minimizes the quantity of data inputs to a reasonable level while maintaining the dataset's integrity to the greatest extent feasible [20]. It's often employed at the data preprocessing step, and there are a variety of dimensionality reduction algorithms to choose from, including the following:

- Principal component analysis

Principal component analysis (PCA) is a dimensionality reduction approach that uses feature extraction to eliminate redundancies and compress datasets [18]. This approach creates a new data representation via a linear transformation, resulting in a collection of "principal components." The direction that maximizes the dataset's variance is the first principal component. While the second main component similarly finds the largest variance in the data, it is entirely unrelated to the first, providing a direction that is perpendicular to the first. This process is repeated for as many dimensions as there are, with the next main component being the direction orthogonal to the previous components with the largest variation [18].

- Singular value decomposition

Similar to PCA, singular value decomposition (SVD) is a technique for reducing noise and compressing data, such as picture files [20].

- Autoencoders

Autoencoders use neural networks to compress data before recreating a new representation of the input data. "Encoding" refers to the stage from the input layer to the hidden layer, whereas "decoding" refers to the stage from the hidden layer to the output layer[20].

6.5 Reinforcement Learning Algorithms

Reinforcement learning (RL) is a machine learning discipline that deals with decision-making and motor control. It investigates how an agent may learn to attain objectives in a complicated and unpredictable environment [2]. The computer uses trial and error to find a solution to the problem. Artificial intelligence is given either incentives or penalties for the actions it takes in order to accomplish what the programmer desires. Its purpose is to increase the overall prize as much as possible [2].

Despite the fact that the designer establishes the reward policy—that is, the game's rules—he provides the model with no tips or ideas for how to complete the game. Starting with completely random trials and progressing to complex strategies and superhuman abilities, it's up to the model to find out how to do the job in order to maximize the reward. Reinforcement learning is currently the most effective technique to hint machine creativity by utilizing the power of search and numerous trials.

The advantages of using RL are as follows:

1. It is a broad term that covers any problem that requires a series of decisions, such as operating a robot's motors so that it may run and leap, making business decisions such as pricing and inventory management, or playing video games and board games.
2. It concentrates on the entire issue. Machine learning algorithms are typically built to excel at certain subtasks, with little regard for the overall picture. RL, on the other hand, does not break the problem down into subproblems; instead, it focuses on maximizing the long-term payoff. It has a clear objective, understands how to achieve it, and can trade short-term gains for long-term gains.
3. It is not necessary to do a separate data collecting process. In RL, training data is gathered by the agent's direct contact with the environment. The learning agent's experience is the training data, not a separate set of data that must be provided to the algorithm. This relieves the supervisor in charge of the training process of a large amount of work.
4. It works in a fast-paced, unpredictable setting. Inherently adaptable, RL algorithms are designed to respond to changes in the environment. Unlike typical machine learning techniques, time is important in RL, and the experience that the agent gathers is not dispersed independently and identically. The learning is intrinsically adaptable since the dimension of time is firmly buried in the mechanics of RL.

Reinforcement learning is often employed in robots, gaming, and navigation. The program uses reinforcement learning to figure out which activities result in the most rewards through trial and error [24].

The agent (the learner or decision-maker), the environment (everything the agent interacts with), and actions are the three main components of this sort of learning (what the agent can do). The agent's goal is to select activities that maximize the predicted reward over a set period of time. By adhering to a sound policy, the agent will be able to achieve the goal much more quickly. There is a task or an activity that must be taught or mastered. If the model successfully completes the task, it is rewarded; if it fails, it is penalized. The challenge with reinforcement learning is determining what kinds of rewards and punishments are appropriate for the model. Based on each data point, these algorithms take an action and then learn how well the decision was. The algorithm adapts its method over time in order to improve its learning and attain the greatest reward.

The computer interacts with its surroundings in reinforcement learning by performing actions a1, a2, and so on. These activities have an impact on the environment, which leads to the machine obtaining scalar rewards (or penalties) r1 and r2. The machine's purpose is to learn to operate in such a manner that it maximizes

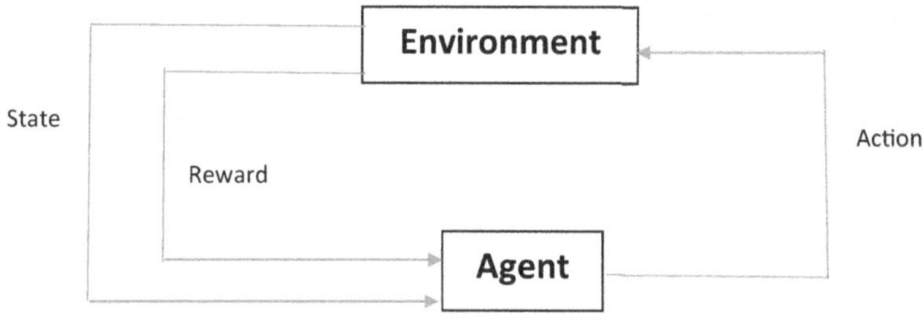

Fig. 6.7 The scenario of reinforcement learning

future rewards (and minimizes future penalties) throughout the course of its existence.

Although distinct elements of the issue and solution are frequently emphasized, the basic problems investigated in these domains are often theoretically similar, and the answers are the same.

Based on each data point, these algorithms take an action and then learn how well the decision was (Fig. 6.7).

- Agent: A supposed being that performs acts in a given environment in exchange for a monetary payment.
- Environment (e) is a situation that agent must deal with.
- Reward (R): An instant monetary reward provided to an agent for completing a specified activity or assignment.
- State (s): Current situation returned by the environment.
- Policy (P): A technique that the agent employs to choose the next action depending on the present condition.
- Value (V): This is the predicted long-term return, discounted from the short-term gain.
- Value function: This function defines the overall amount of reward for a certain state. Beginning with that state, it is an agent to be expected.
- Environmental model: This simulates environmental behavior. It assists you in drawing conclusions and predicting how the environment will react.
- Model-based techniques: Model-based methods are a type of method for tackling reinforcement learning challenges.
- Action value (Q) or Q value: The terms value and Q value are pretty similar. The only distinction is that as a current action, it accepts an extra argument.

The agent continues to do the three things (take action, change state or remain in the same state, and receive feedback) and, as a result of the activities, learns and explores the world.

By using the Markov decision process, the problem in RL will be formulated and presented.

A finite number of states and actions are assumed in Markov decision process problems (MDPs). Each time the agent observes a state and takes a step, it incurs intermediate costs that must be kept to a minimum (or, in the inverse scenario, rewards to be maximized). The cost and successor state are solely determined by the present condition and the action taken. Based on the uncertainty we have about the environment in which the search takes place, successor generation might be probabilistic. An action, for example, may occasionally fail to produce the desired target state, thus remaining in the present state with a tiny probability.

Reinforcement learning characteristics:

- There is no supervisor, but simply a number or a signal of reward.
- Making decisions in a sequential order.
- In reinforcement issues, time is critical.
- Feedback is never immediate; it is always delayed.
- The data that the agent gets is determined by its activities.

Reinforcement learning types.

There are two sorts of reinforcement learning methods: positive and negative.

- Positive

It is described as an occurrence that occurs as a result of certain actions. It improves the strength and frequency of the behavior and has a beneficial influence on the agent's actions.

This sort of reinforcement aids in maximizing performance and maintaining change for a longer length of time. However, too much reinforcement might lead to state over-optimization, which can have an impact on the outcome.

- Negative

Negative reinforcement is defined as behavior strengthening that happens as a result of a negative circumstance that should have been avoided or halted. It assists you in determining the minimal level of performance. The disadvantage of this strategy is that it just gives enough to fulfill the basic behavior requirements.

A reinforcement learning algorithm may be implemented in three ways:

1. Value-based: The value-based method is concerned with determining the optimal value function, or the maximum value at a given state under any policy. As a result, the agent anticipates a long-term return in any of the policy's states.
2. Policy-based: Without employing the value function, a policy-based method is used to discover the best policy for maximal future benefits. In this technique, the agent strives to implement a policy in which each step's activity contributes to the future reward being maximized.

There are two sorts of policies in the policy-based approach: The first one is deterministic strategy, in which the policy produces the same action in any state, and the second one is stochastic strategy, in which the resulting action is determined by chance.

3. Model-based: A virtual model of the world is generated for the model-based method, and the agent explores it to understand it. Because each environment's

model representation is distinct, there is no specific solution or methodology for this method.

RL algorithms are divided into two categories: model-based and model-free.

The fundamental advantage of having a model is that it allows the agent to plan by thinking ahead, visualizing what would happen if they made a variety of different choices, and openly choosing among them. Agents can then synthesize the outcomes of their foresight into a learned policy.

The fundamental disadvantage is that the agent rarely has access to a ground-truth representation of the environment. In this instance, if an agent wishes to utilize a model, it must learn it entirely via experience, which presents a number of difficulties. The most significant difficulty is that the agent can exploit model bias, resulting in an agent that performs well in the learned model but acts sub-optimally (or horribly) in the actual world. Model learning is essentially difficult, so even putting in a lot of effort, putting in a lot of time, and computing power might not be enough.

- Model-based (algorithms which use a model): An algorithm that estimates the best policy using the transition function (and the reward function).
- Model-free (algorithms which don't use a model): An algorithm that calculates the best policy without utilizing or predicting the environment's dynamics (transition and reward functions).

One of the most famous model-free algorithms used in reinforcement learning is Q-learning.

- Q-Learning

The Q in Q-learning stands for quality; it is a type of reinforcement learning that does not need the use of a model [21]. It may also be thought of as an asynchronous dynamic programming technique (DP). It enables agents to learn how to operate optimally in Markovian domains by exposing them to consequences of actions rather than forcing them to develop domain mappings [21]. Q-learning is a learner who does not follow the rules. That is, it learns the value of the best policy without relying on the agent's behaviors. An on-policy learner, on the other hand, learns the value of the policy being carried out by the agent, including the exploration phases, and it will choose the best policy possible, taking into consideration the policy's exploration.

6.6 Deep Learning

Deep learning is a technique and subset of machine learning that trains computers to do what people do naturally: learn by doing [32]. Deep learning is a critical component of self-driving automobiles, allowing them to recognize a stop sign or discriminate between a pedestrian and a lamppost. It enables voice control in consumer electronics such as phones, tablets, televisions, and hands-free speakers. Deep learning has gotten a lot of press recently, and for good cause. It's accomplishing accomplishments that were previously unattainable [32].

A computer model learns to execute categorization tasks directly from pictures, text, or sound in deep learning. Deep learning models can attain state-of-the-art accuracy, even surpassing human performance in some cases. Models are trained utilizing a huge quantity of labeled data and multilayer neural network topologies.

Deep learning achieves better recognition accuracy than ever before. This enables consumer electronics to satisfy user expectations, which is vital for safety-sensitive applications such as self-driving cars. Deep learning has progressed to the point that it now surpasses humans in some tasks, such as categorizing objects in photographs [32, 44].

Large volumes of labeled data are required for deep learning. It also needs a significant amount of computational power. The parallel design of high-performance graphical user interface is ideal for deep learning. When used in conjunction with clusters or cloud computing, this allows development teams to cut deep learning network training time from weeks to hours or less [32].

Deep learning models are sometimes referred to as deep neural networks since most deep learning approaches employ neural network designs [23].The number of hidden layers in a neural network is commonly referred to as "deep." Deep neural networks can have up to 150 hidden layers, whereas traditional neural networks only have 2–3.

Large amounts of labeled data and neural network topologies that learn features directly from the data without the requirement for manual feature extraction are used to train deep learning models.

Figure 6.8 demonstrates deep neural networks.

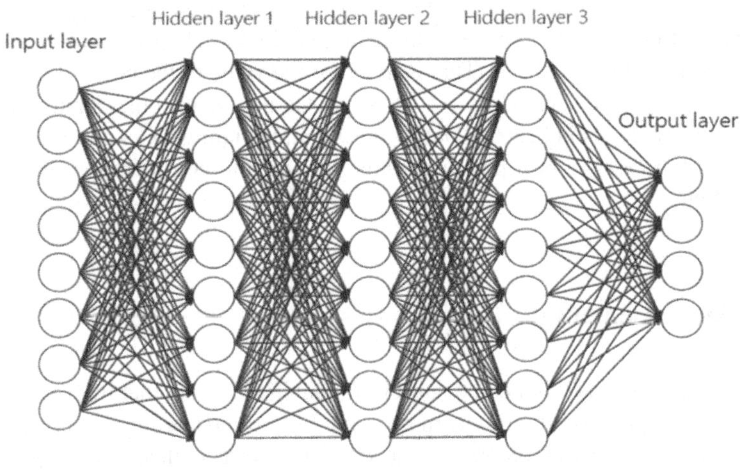

Fig. 6.8 Deep neural network

Convolutional neural networks are one of the most often used deep neural network types (CNN or ConvNet) which learns directly from data, eliminating the need for manual feature extraction. A CNN employs 2D convolutional layers to combine learned characteristics with incoming data, making it well-suited to processing 2D data like images. CNNs are very effective for recognizing objects, people, and sceneries in photos by looking for patterns. Nonimage data, such as audio, time series, and signal data, may also be classified using them. CNNs are used extensively in applications that need object identification and computer vision, including as self-driving cars and facial recognition [37].

The use of CNNs for deep learning is common for three reasons:

1. CNNs eliminate the requirement for manual feature extraction since the CNN learns the features directly.
2. CNNs yield very accurate recognition results.
3. CNNs may be retrained for new recognition tasks, allowing you to extend the capabilities of current networks.

CNNs are an important technology in medical imaging because they can visually discover image defects by examining hundreds of pathology reports. A convolutional neural network can include tens or hundreds of layers, each of which learns to recognize distinct picture characteristics. At various resolutions, filters are applied to each training image, and the result of each convolved image is utilized as the input to the next layer. The filters can start with very basic qualities like brightness and edges and progress to more complicated attributes that describe the item uniquely [49].

A CNN, like other neural networks, has an input layer, an output layer, but a huge number of hidden layers in between.

These layers conduct operations on the data with the goal of learning data-specific characteristics. Convolution, activation or ReLU, and pooling are three of the most popular layers.

- Convolution passes the input pictures through a series of convolutional filters, each of which activates different aspects of the image.

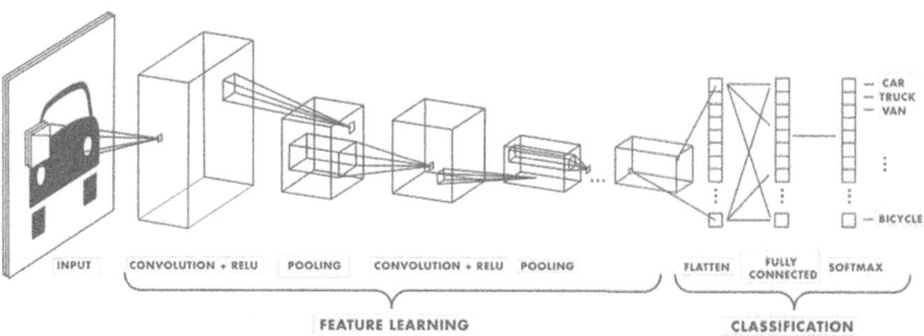

Fig. 6.9 Example of training image

- Rectified linear unit (ReLU) or activation: By mapping negative values to zero and keeping positive values, it is possible to train quicker and more effectively. Because only the active characteristics are carried on into the next layer, this is frequently referred to as activation.
- Pooling reduces the number of parameters that the network must learn by conducting nonlinear downsampling on the output.

These actions are performed several times over, with each layer learning to recognize distinct characteristics.

Figure 6.9 shows example of training image by a network with several convolutional layers with the most three popular layers, and the result of each convolved image is utilized as the input to the next layer.

A CNN has neurons with weights and biases, just like a typical neural network. During the training phase, the model learns these values and updates them with each new training sample. In the case of CNNs, however, all hidden neurons in a layer have the identical weights and bias values. This suggests that all hidden neurons are detecting the same feature in various parts of the picture, such as an edge or a blob. As a result, the network is tolerant to picture object translation. A network trained to detect autos, for example, will be able to do so regardless of where the car appears in the image.

The design of a CNN turns to categorization after learning characteristics in several layers. The layer after that is a fully connected layer that produces a vector with N dimensions, where N is the number of classes that the network can predict. The probabilities for each class of every picture being categorized are contained in this vector. The classification output is provided by the last layer of the CNN design, which employs a classification layer.

References

1. Arulkumaran K, Deisenroth MP, Brundage M, Bharath AA (2017) Deep reinforcement learning: a brief survey. IEEE Signal Process Mag 34(6):26–38
2. Bar-Gad I, Morris G, Bergman H (2003) Information processing, dimensionality reduction and reinforcement learning in the basal ganglia. Prog Neurobiol 71(6):439–473
3. Bortoloti FD, de Oliveira E, Ciarelli PM (2021) Supervised kernel density estimation K-means. Expert Syst Appl 168:114350
4. Buşoniu L, Babuška R, Schutter BD (2010) Multi-agent reinforcement learning: an overview. Innovations in multi-agent systems and applications-1:183–221
5. Caruana R, Niculescu-Mizil A (2006) An empirical comparison of supervised learning algorithms. Paper presented at the proceedings of the 23rd international conference on machine learning
6. Celebi ME, Aydin K (2016) Unsupervised learning algorithms. Springer
7. Cios KJ, Swiniarski RW, Pedrycz W, Kurgan LA (2007) Unsupervised learning: association rules. Paper presented at the Data Mining
8. Cunningham P, Cord M, Delany SJ (2008) Supervised learning machine learning techniques for multimedia. Springer, pp 21–49

9. Cuzzolin F, Morelli A, Cirstea B, Sahakian BJ (2020) Knowing me, knowing you: theory of mind in AI. Psychol Med 50(7):1057–1061
10. Diaz-Rozo J, Bielza C, Larranaga P (2020) Machine-tool condition monitoring with Gaussian mixture models-based dynamic probabilistic clustering. Eng Appl Artif Intell 89:103434
11. Dike HU, Zhou Y, Deveerasetty KK, Wu Q (2018) Unsupervised learning based on artificial neural network: a review. Paper presented at the 2018 IEEE international conference on cyborg and bionic systems (CBS)
12. Dimiduk DM, Holm EA, Niezgoda SR (2018) Perspectives on the impact of machine learning, deep learning, and artificial intelligence on materials, processes, and structures engineering. Integrat Mat Manufact Innovat 7(3):157–172
13. Dunjko V, Briegel HJ (2018) Machine learning & artificial intelligence in the quantum domain: a review of recent progress. Rep Prog Phys 81(7):074001. https://doi.org/10.1088/1361-6633/aab406
14. Enrici I, Bara BG, Adenzato M (2019) Theory of mind, pragmatics and the brain: converging evidence for the role of intention processing as a core feature ofhuman communication. Pragmat Cognition 26(1):5–38
15. Geurts P, Irrthum A, Wehenkel L (2009) Supervised learning with decision tree-based methods in computational and systems biology. Mol BioSyst 5(12):1593–1605
16. Haldorai A, Kandaswamy U (2019) Supervised machine learning techniques in intelligent network handovers. In: Intelligent Spectrum Handovers in Cognitive Radio Networks. Springer, pp 135–154
17. Harrington P (2012) Machine learning in action. Simon and Schuster
18. Hasan BMS, Abdulazeez AM (2021) A review of principal component analysis algorithm for dimensionality reduction. J Soft Computi Data Mining 2(1):20–30
19. Hassani H, Silva ES, Unger S, TajMazinani M, Mac Feely S (2020) Artificial intelligence (AI) or intelligence augmentation (IA): what is the future? Ai 1(2):143–155
20. Hurtik P, Molek V, Perfilieva I (2020) Novel dimensionality reduction approach for unsupervised learning on small datasets. Pattern Recogn 103:107291
21. Jang B, Kim M, Harerimana G, Kim JW (2019) Q-learning algorithms: a comprehensive classification and applications. IEEE Access 7:133653–133667
22. Kaur D, Sahdev SL, Sharma D, Siddiqui L (2020) Banking 4.0:'the influence of artificial intelligence on the Banking Industry & how AI is changing the face of modern day banks'. Inter J Manag 11(6)
23. Kriegeskorte N, Golan T (2019) Neural network models and deep learning. Curr Biol 29(7):R231–R236
24. Lee JA, Verleysen M (2007) Nonlinear dimensionality reduction, vol 1. Springer
25. Likas A, Vlassis N, Verbeek JJ (2003) The global k-means clustering algorithm. Pattern Recogn 36(2):451–461
26. Lu H, Li Y, Chen M, Kim H, Serikawa S (2018) Brain intelligence: go beyond artificial intelligence. Mobile Networks Applicat 23(2):368–375. https://doi.org/10.1007/s11036-017-0932-8
27. Mitchell M (2005) Self-awareness and control in decentralized systems. Paper presented at the Aaai spring symposium: metacognition in computation
28. Nasteski V (2017) An overview of the supervised machine learning methods. Horizons b 4:51–62
29. Nazari Z, Kang D, Asharif MR, Sung Y, Ogawa S (2015) A new hierarchical clustering algorithm. Paper presented at the 2015 international conference on intelligent informatics and biomedical sciences (ICIIBMS)
30. Nilsson NJ, Nilsson NJ (1998) Artificial intelligence: a new synthesis. Morgan Kaufmann
31. Omran MG, Engelbrecht AP, Salman A (2007) An overview of clustering methods. Intelligent Data Analy 11(6):583–605
32. Ongsulee P (2017) Artificial intelligence, machine learning and deep learning. Paper presented at the 2017 15th international conference on ICT and knowledge engineering (ICT&KE)

33. Ossowska A, Kusiak A, Swietlik D (2022) Artificial intelligence in dentistry-narrative review. Int J Environ Res Public Health 19(6). https://doi.org/10.3390/ijerph19063449
34. Rajaram NS (1990) Artificial intelligence: a technology review. ISA Trans 29(1):1–3. https://doi.org/10.1016/0019-0578(90)90023-e
35. Saravanan R, Sujatha P (2018) A state of art techniques on machine learning algorithms: a perspective of supervised learning approaches in data classification. Paper presented at the 2018 second international conference on intelligent computing and control systems (ICICCS)
36. Sathya R, Abraham A (2013) Comparison of supervised and unsupervised learning algorithms for pattern classification. Inter J Advanc Res Artif Intellig 2(2):34–38
37. Schmidhuber J (2015) Deep learning in neural networks: an overview. Neural Netw 61:85–117
38. Schwenker F, Trentin E (2014) Pattern classification and clustering: a review of partially supervised learning approaches. Pattern Recogn Lett 37:4–14
39. Sejnowski TJ (2020) The unreasonable effectiveness of deep learning in artificial intelligence. Proc Natl Acad Sci 117(48):30033–30038
40. Sharma R, Kim M, Gupta A (2022) Motor imagery classification in brain-machine interface with machine learning algorithms: classical approach to multi-layer perceptron model. Biomed Signal Process Cont 71:103101
41. Shinners L, Aggar C, Grace S, Smith S (2020) Exploring healthcare professionals' understanding and experiences of artificial intelligence technology use in the delivery of healthcare: an integrative review. Health Informatics J 26(2):1225–1236. https://doi.org/10.1177/1460458219874641
42. Shmilovici A (2009) Support vector machines. In: Data mining and knowledge discovery handbook. Springer, pp 231–247
43. Sinaga KP, Yang M-S (2020) Unsupervised K-means clustering algorithm. IEEE Access 8:80716–80727
44. Skansi S (2018) Introduction to deep learning: from logical calculus to artificial intelligence. Springer
45. Sutton RS (1992) Introduction: the challenge of reinforcement learning. In: Reinforcement learning. Springer, pp 1–3
46. Sutton RS, Barto AG (2018) Reinforcement learning: an introduction. MIT press
47. Wang X, Lin X, Dang X (2020) Supervised learning in spiking neural networks: a review of algorithms and evaluations. Neural Netw 125:258–280
48. Wang Z, Keane PA, Chiang M, Cheung CY, Wong TY, Ting DSW (2020) Artificial intelligence and deep learning in ophthalmology. Artif Intell Med:1–34
49. Yasaka K, Akai H, Kunimatsu A, Kiryu S, Abe O (2018) Deep learning with convolutional neural network in radiology. Jpn J Radiol 36(4):257–272
50. Yürüşen NY, Uzunoğlu B, Talayero AP, Estopiñán AL (2021) Apriori and K-means algorithms of machine learning for spatio-temporal solar generation balancing. Renew Energy 175:702–717

Chapter 7
AI in Oral Health and Oral Imaging

7.1 Impact of AI on the Global Health: Role of AI in Public Health Dentistry

Artificial intelligence is most likely to become a building block of future dentistry, promising order-of-magnitude improvements in disease detection and treatment. The extent to which our understanding of the impact the technology may have on people, systems, and societies is currently unknown, particularly regarding the domain of application of the technology in low-resource settings.

Artificial intelligence (AI) has proved a cutting-edge technology in detecting, diagnostics, and treating oral diseases. Topol [1] suggested that deep learning, a subset of artificial neural network-based machine learning, has enabled impressive performance consistent with trained practitioners' interpretation of x-ray images, photos, symptoms, and habits [1].

Contemporaneous advances in IT in a large number of underdeveloped and developing countries (otherwise known as low- to middle-income countries) imply that artificial intelligence (AI) is likely to hold the key to future global health, given its capacity to cope with arising challenges and ensure sustainable success of developmental objectives in the fields of health and prevention.

We evidence a heated debate about emerging AI-governed health interventions, applications, and approaches compared to traditional procedures usually undertaken to achieve informed and ethical decision-making. Many health issues common to LMICs have been deployed lately, interventions primarily focusing on infectious diseases, such as tuberculosis and malaria. The artificial intelligence concept varies in types.

However, numerous forms of machine learning or signal processing are predominantly applied, frequently in synergy with other methods, principally signal-to-process. It is reported that there are four AI-driven health interventions, classified in separate categories: (1) diagnostics, (2) patient mortality risk assessment, (3)

K. Shaikh et al., *Artificial Intelligence in Dentistry*,
https://doi.org/10.1007/978-3-031-19715-4_7

disease outbreak prediction and surveillance, and (4) health policy and planning. However, the majority of literature of global research into the AI-governed intervention in the domain of global health does not account for diverse ethical, administrative, or practical considerations required for large-scale use of AI in the realm of global health.

Although the project of AI-driven health interventions has taken off only recently, it is said to be a promising platform for achieving favorable results in LMICs. In their study of challenges relative to developing and deploying the AI-driven interventions, Nina S. and Brian W. (2020) suggest that AI-driven no matter how specific a particular setting for intervention is, there is a growing need to develop thorough methodological guidelines that will define the scope, the function, and the goals of an AI approach to the global health-care system, taking into consideration all ethical limitations and concerns that might further direct the research agenda in the field [2].

Generally, three application domains are related to AI-based health-care interventions in oral public health. The first one encompasses AI-driven tools used on smartphones or portables. Operated by nonspecialist community health workers (CHWs), based on off-site locations, these typically address traditional oral diseases. As reported by Hosny and Aerts (2019), CHWs may follow AI recommendations to triage patients and identify those requiring immediate treatment [3]. This category of application involves the diagnostics of oral and labial cancer based on photographic images and peripheral blood samples. The advent of pocket diagnostic hardware (ultrasound probes and microscopes) also promises rapid improvements in this domain. Ubiquitous smartphones will allow patients to use AI to design their nutrition and daily routines.

The technology will also enable symptoms self-assessment and cover the advisory aspect during pregnancy or recovery phases, eventually allowing patients to monitor their health, thus facilitating the operation of the health system.

The following application area centers on more specialized medical requirements to hold up decision-making in the clinical environment. AI may be useful among nonspecialized general dental practitioners for more specialized purposes, such as reading diagnostic radiology and pathology images, which will further ensure that specialists are consulted only if the necessity arises. Additionally, AI tools may also offer professional knowledge within a multitude of subspecialties, i.e., in oral oncology, the AI use may allow the oncologist to safely manage tumors in several anatomical sites. In radiotherapy, semi-automation may help provide some advantages. Treatment planning may hasten the delivery of treatment, enhance patient's intake, or permit specialists to focus on other aspects of patient management without additional human resources requirements. Although AI may not directly impact diagnostic tools and therapeutic equipment shortages, embedding AI into equipment planning may help nontechnical practitioners tackle specific issues lacking technical personnel. By chronologically analyzing maintenance data, AI may also preserve long-term operations plans, help professionals predict possible failures, and provide spare parts management.

Finally, AI-based application refers to the domain of population oral health and public agencies' activities aimed at sensing cause-and-effect correlations, proper resource allocating, and finally managing the progression of diseases in epidemics. Advancing data collection is the focus of these applications, i.e., AI-based design provides continuous maintenance of national cancer registries along with several operations that may help reduce operating costs.

AI-based applications in health care are still in the infancy phase, as the majority of the uses are currently in the proof-of-concept stage, necessitating clinical validation through specific procedures and trials. The methods used generally do not allow proper data interpretation, thus hindering the prediction of failures and critical assessment of the results. In addition, the adverse circumstance that data used to train AI models are gathered within high-income countries (HICs) is hampering the full implementation of AI. The models are limited to several elements, such as some disease demographics, etc. Nonuniform and unsteady statistical data analysis and quality control result in inconsistencies that allow for errors producing models that prevent establishing generalizations, etc. Apprehension exists regarding certain ethical concerns, e.g., patients' data privacy breach as a third entity is introduced into the patient-doctor relationship. From the aspect of the regulation, possible medical malpractices and liabilities arising from newly established algorithmic decision-making are yet to be formulated. Given that almost all AI tools in health care refer to single-task applications, these are not anticipated to fully substitute health professionals, which helps to lower the expectations.

Introducing AI tools in resource-limited environments poses challenges. Given the diverse needs, disease specificities, as well as those of demographics and standards across low- and middle-income countries (LMICs), specific AI application cases with the most prominent influence need to be identified and acknowledged accordingly.

Context-specific training and validation data are necessary, along with solutions required to be context-specific. The latter primarily refers to the requirement that an automated system be prevented from recommending treatments unaccessible locally or those that are unlawfully expensive. What is more, human factors need to be observed, i.e., competencies, education, and digital literacy of end users. The behavioral aspect relative to raising awareness and confidence in AI systems should also be in focus, as this will let users recognize limitations and accurately read the results. Availability of devices supporting AI applications, e.g., continuous, and steady, Internet throughput, electricity, etc. also need to be assessed. Various digital initiatives have additionally improved the quality of health-care services in low- and middle-income countries. These involve health-care practices supporting technologies such as eHealth and telehealth platforms (telecommunication/mobile health (mHealth)). The highest- performance practices for scaling these digital initiatives in LMICs ambiance have been established based on hands-on experiences. These endeavors could enable a learning environment for related digital AI applications. Some challenging but still adverse factors, such as limited funding and inappropriate and unreliable infrastructure, may stand in AI applications' fast and proper implementation. Integration opportunities could also be considered: for instance, a proper mHealth application designed for patient-doctor distance communication can be upgraded with an AI chatbot to triage patients before the consultation.

Some questions have been raised concerning the value of the implementation of AI in LMICs since it is primarily a basic infrastructure that necessitates investments [4]. AI-governed interventions should not be assessed in isolation, nor should they be attributed to cure-all capacities [4]. "Although sizable initial investments may be required, the marginal cost of providing an existing AI software service to one more user is minuscule, giving it economical scalability" [3] as the existing digital technologies may also offer to provide proper utilization of AI application [3]. Finally, the incentive for AI in health-care interventions within LMICs should be managed entirely by local stakeholders in charge of funding. At present, AI literacy is presupposed in global health educational programs, the trend that will undoubtedly continue in the future, aimed to raise awareness of its capacities and possible drawbacks. Promoting the AI concept locally will be of utmost importance, with the capability to be promoted through free educational online programs. The incorporation of AI will also need to rely on regulatory frameworks, which need to be adjusted to allow effective implementation of the concept, e.g., the training of local health professionals may be extended to involve screening and diagnosing noncommunicable diseases (NCDs) [5]. Two crucial aspects to be identified to introduce AI into LMICs are investments and obtaining data on the impact of AI solutions. As the existing tensions between social groups (the rich-the poor) have been additionally increased by an uneven distribution of access to digital technologies, AI could be a mediator capable of mitigating the differences as a socially responsible technology available to all social classes.

7.2 Applications of Artificial Intelligence (AI) in Public Health Dentistry

- **Dental AI Applications**

AI in health care is booming, with the traditional dentistry sector evolving and being gradually transformed into digital dentistry. As AI technology rapidly advances every day, we are expected to witness a growing impact of AI in dentistry in the future as it allows enormous benefits for both dental clinics and patients. Furthermore, current research suggests that AI might seriously affect the job markets, as it will replace or repurpose certain professions [6]. The introduction of AI tools in dentistry reduces both human errors and costs.

AI in dentistry functions as a complementary tool that deals with vast amounts of health data (HD). Algorithms and IT applications approximate human cognition in analyzing complex data. The main goal is to analyze the arduous task that a human would otherwise be solved exclusively. AI solutions have been increasingly used to support doctors' decisions in diagnostic suggestions, therapeutic protocols, personalized medicine, patient monitoring, and predicting and tracking epidemiological diseases' expansion. The fields of AI application vary from health emergencies, prevention, and treatment techniques to the analytics of patient outcomes.

In this context, AI is expected to provide additional support to practitioners by allowing the transfer of knowledge from basic and clinical research to health professionals and their attempts to search for the best approaches for their patients. The gap between in vitro findings and the straight way into (routine) clinical therapy needs to be overcome to benefit a larger patient population and be made accessible to underdeveloped countries [7]. In addition to this, AI is expected to bridge the gaps between medicine and dentistry to explore and interpret the influence of general disease patterns on oral health.

Apart from generally accelerating the workflows, AI is constantly achieving breakthroughs, thus allowing practitioners to utilize novel and innovative solutions in several aspects of their work. For example, AI-driven custom-designed orthodontic treatments are a recent innovation. However, advanced tools also focus on diagnostic records of virtual IOPAs/RVGs, 3D scans, and cone-beam computed tomography. The field of restorative and prosthetic medicine has made a step forward with the application of computer-aided designs and computer-aided production technology for a precision fit, which can have a vital impact on orofacial and craniofacial prosthetics. From that perspective, AI can have an essential role in all stages of the dental workflow, from endodontics to apex location dentistry. Apart from upgrading dentistry as a field, dental AI will significantly affect implantology for making precise surgical guides and determining cortical bone thickness.

As evidence suggests, AI-based virtual dental assistants can carry out tasks that would sometimes require an entire team of people with different skills and backgrounds. Even though such tasks are various, AI applications perform many tasks with higher precision and efficiency than humans. It primarily refers to operational tasks such as booking or coordinating regular appointments, notification to patients and dentists about checkups, clinical diagnosis assistance, and treatment agenda. In addition, AI allows patients to participate in the global health-care system more personally, especially if they willingly provide data of their health habits and conditions. Patients can also be actively involved in self-monitoring and self-management. As AI has an option to "learn" from the collected data, there are mechanisms to overcome the disadvantages of on-off medicine (e.g., periodontal disease).

If there is continuous AI supervision of a patient's health record, a more comprehensive and accurate understanding of the patient's health condition is available. With such an approach, both diagnostic and treatment costs can be decreased, thus making health-care systems less busy and overburdened. From a more global perspective, AI can also help solve the problem of workforce shortages, in that context complying with the World Health Organization (WHO) Sustainable Development Goals.

Since the 2000s, a global scientific focus has been shifted to various aspects of artificial intelligence. Even though there is unambiguous evidence that AI systems have brought success to various academic and business fields, much more needs to be done to prevent and promote the population's health in terms of AI applications. In other words, we need to address how AI solutions can act as a social predictor that would have a more significant impact on the actual outcomes. As AI applications have been reported to match or outperform humans in various domains, it is

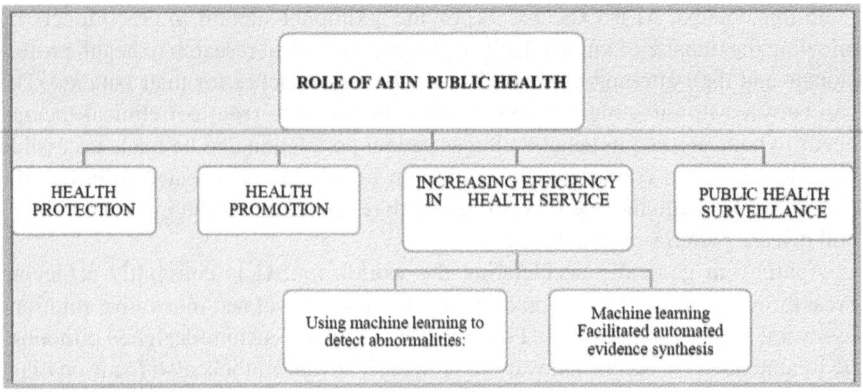

Fig. 7.1 Role of artificial intelligence in public health [8]

yet to be seen what essential benefits, on a global scale, AI brings, especially when compared to practical implications stemming from research studies coming from academic communities (Fig. 7.1).

One possible utilization of the artificial intelligence concept in health promotion is analyzing datasets for almost real-time surveillance and oral disease detection, e.g., screening and identifying suspected changed mucosa undergoing premalignant and malignant alterations or diagnosing and treating oral cavity lesions. AI has the potential to showcase images that document the slightest changes, measured in pixels, that would not be possible to notice by the traditional examination technique. When the dental health-care professional is unavailable, and there is a health emergency, AI can assist by providing E-assistance (tele-assistance). Behavior patterns and risk profiles designed by AI algorithms can be utilized for individually tailored health advice. Recently, there has been an increased interest in computer-aided decision-making in this field, probably due to improved digital literacy in the general population. For instance, it would be useful to alert a dental practitioner about any medical condition or oral habit that might predict genetic oral disease risk in a large population.

It is not an overstatement to say that artificial intelligence can significantly increase the efficiency of health services in numerous ways, some of the critical ones being as follows:

Using Machine Learning to Detect Abnormalities

Clinical decision support system may effectively provide valuable medical professionals valuable data, thus improving health outcomes for dual patients and the general population. Ultimately, AI has proven its usefulness in providing high-precision images in the field of medicine. There is evidence that AI-powered artificial neural networks can detect signs of oral cancer and other conditions with the same accuracy and reliability as human radiologists. In addition, AI proves support to a dentist to spot early signs of disease.

Machine Learning-Facilitated Automated Evidence Synthesis
The traditional procedure of entering any structured information in the health system appears to be a time-consuming work. However, the process has been drastically facilitated by the introduction of voice recognition and the application of AI programs to classify and excerpt information from the scanned paperwork. It should also be stressed that its interactive character allows health-care professionals to process more data than human assistants would generally more efficiently and reliably [8].

- **AI and Dental Clinic Management**

The roles of AI as a constative element in the public oral health upgrade and significance are best shown in dental clinics' management or general operations. Scheduling patient appointments is one of such aspects, and newly appointed assistants can be easily trained to perform such tasks more efficiently and productively.

Another aspect of AI smart scheduling appointments is best demonstrated in doctor-patient communication. To arrange systematic contacts of patients based on their appointment preference and match patients with an available position for arranging to schedule proprietary algorithms to identify the ideal patients, the program automates scheduling existing patients with voice, text, or even video. It will also initiate the ideal marketing campaign to convert new patients. Another advanced aspect of AI in scheduling appointments is the possibility to track and optimize patient appointments so that it allows to "proactively schedule unfinished treatment and launch new-patient marketing campaigns based on profit maximization algorithms" [9]. Such optimization is achieved by machine learning programs that can interface with dental practice software. As far as patient's general queries are concerned, all simple questions can be easily handled by AI. In contrast, more complex ones can be directed to the practitioner for further processing. The neural network can also mine data and detect periods of decreased productivity to help determine the most effective marketing campaign. The variety of possibilities within this algorithm allows management officers to see cancellations or supervise the available appointments easily. In contrast, deep learning techniques allow searching patient records for the most profitable patient treatment. In that sense, assistants spend less time dealing with prescriptions post-op and can act more readily before the actual appointment if there is an emergency with a patient to be recognized. In addition to this, and for the more significant benefit of patients, AI can support the dental health-care professional in terms of any relevant medical history or allergies that the patient may have. Patients who are on tobacco or smoking cessation programs, for example, can utilize AI to set up necessary reminders.

In rare cases when a doctor is not available, AI can serve as a helping hand, as it can store different information related to a patient's health conditions. Apart from documentation and scientific coding, it can hold and retain patient's databases, help monitor patients' orders, observe health situations in addition to preventive measures, etc.

With the big data, including electronic health records, digital radiographs, and longitudinal follow-up data, it will be possible to establish a reliable source for training the Al system. Predictions will be significantly improved with a better understanding of the patient's condition drawing upon vast data. This implies that the Al scientific data library will keep itself updated with the current literature knowledge in the field, as it can learn from the scientific database.

Unlike other (traditional) methods of operations in dental clinics, AI software enables us to design a comprehensive virtual database for every patient, which can be easily highlighted and accessible at the same time [10]. For example, voice recognition and interactive interphases enable the software to help the dentist perform different tasks effortlessly. As the AI software can retrieve all necessary data from the database and present it to the dentist much faster and more efficiently than a human counterpart (e.g., collecting all essential dental records, extraoral photographs, and radiographs necessary for diagnosing any dental condition), any dental intervention becomes more reliable. Because of its unique ability to learn, the AI system can be "trained" to perform many other functions. For instance, it can be integrated with imaging systems like MRI and CBCT to identify slight deviations from normalcy that could have gone unnoticed to the human eye.

On the other hand, however, artificial intelligence is still growing in the dental field. It is not yet that advanced that could duly replace human's skills and competence. If perceived as a complementary technology, AI can assist in numerous dental operations or help raise more awareness of oral and maxillofacial diseases while encouraging patients to schedule for preliminary treatment. Even though at its infancy, AI has produced staggering solutions that might drastically change dental procedures in the future. Computer systems with human-level intelligence (or higher) will change the world as we know it, thus affecting our lives. What remains as a currently debatable issue is the general concern in what way and to what extent AI could be integrated into practice, as it is a general standpoint that AI cannot act as a complete substitute to a dentist, since the clinical trial is not only about diagnoses, but it also includes correlating with clinical findings and imparting personalized patient care. Although AI can be utilized as a handy and quick solution in many ways, some of which have been mentioned in the text, the final decisions need to be made exclusively by dentists, as dentistry is a multidisciplinary approach that needs to consider numerous specific elements related to human health.

- **AI and the Financial Aspect of Dental Care**

The financial aspect of dental care is another segment of dentistry in which AI proves to be highly beneficial. Dental AI makes the dental process more transparent for both payer and provider when dealing with the same documentation. In other words, dentists who practice the use of AI in their clinical workflow will be able to understand if there is proper, evidence-based documentation and whether it aligns with the insurer's policies. For example, if there is a need to photograph broken cusp when it is not apparent in a radiograph, AI systems can make the necessity for a picture. In that way, misinterpretations of clinical guidelines are minimized, and care providers become quite aware of the objective measures used by payers. Of course, clinicians reviewing claims need to be consistent when applying standards. If inconsistency in claims review occurs, it is usually due to two factors:

inter-clinician variability and sampling of claims for review. As for inter-clinician variability, it is expectable that the more clinicians review the same claim or radiograph, the more potentially different viewpoints we get. Various providers might propose multiple treatment plans for a single patient. Different perspectives of the same situation may occur due to previous skills or training, experience, or even fatigue of the dental provider. As research suggests, AI can help provide reliable and precise measurements that support or recommend each claim without unnecessary subjective estimates, which may vary (i.e., whether the amount of missing tooth structure is 40% or 50%). In such cases, dental consultants will consider outputs from the AI analysis before making the final decision [11].

What can be done to prevent inconsistency in claims review? Indeed, as it can affect provider satisfaction, arouse tensions between payers and providers, and even influence the increase in appeal rates, inconsistency in claims review should be carefully dealt with, with significant AI assistance in that matter. Radiographs can be reviewed with standardized measurements on AI systems, and it can be documented that a tooth needs further intervention according to clinical guidelines.

Recent research suggests that AI-enhanced claims review will ultimately lower costs since every time an appeal is filed or a claim is resubmitted, it increases costs to both parties. Another reason inconsistency in claims adjudication occurs is the fact that only a small number get processed due to a shortage of dental consultants. In those cases, although two separate benefit claims for the same diagnosis can be submitted, payment will be received for only one share. The reason behind this is that a denial of benefit payment may have been warranted in both cases, however, if the approved claim was not assessed by clinical review and therefore benefited by default. Since this situation might obviously provoke a revolt in both providers and patients, AI support can be beneficial as it can process all reviewable claims signaling those claims that do not meet the prescribed standards for the claims that can be approved. In both scenarios, the process is conducted consistently and efficiently [12].

This specific application of AI in claims review brings about numerous benefits for patients. As the system will bring fewer patient appeals and lessen the number of surprise denials, the system's transparency will be improved. If used regularly, the AI system will ensure validity and confidence with patients for their prospective dental benefits and treatment plans. Consequently, the improved efficiency in reviewing claims will speed reimbursement and lessen the administrative costs from payers. This will reflect the slower growth of premiums for patients and employers.

Another significant benefit of the AI system in dental clinics in terms of financial aspect is instant predetermination, as nowadays, many dental payers offer predeterminations or pre-estimates. In costly procedures, payers prefer predetermination to identify contractual limitations or exclusions that apply to a proposed treatment plan, including certain exclusions or limitations to the proposed plan. Although some plan details can be offered on project player websites, additional time is needed to create and deliver a clinical review, so turnaround times for payers increase to 2 or 3 weeks. Dental AI is expected to transform this process soon.

AI adoption has already commenced for internal claims review and in provider offices. As the main goal for providers and payers is to provide the best experience for patients, and AI potentially brings more clarity and reliability for patients, all parties involved in the process will rely on AI solutions. Finally, the AI paradigm reduces financial uncertainty for patients and helps general dentistry find solutions to resolving delays that can discourage medically necessary treatments.

7.3 AI in Preventive Dentistry

- **Artificial Intelligence in Infection Surveillance and Prevention**

Besides its application in dental diagnostics, treatment, and management, artificial intelligence has demonstrated tremendous potential in infection surveillance and prevention.

The surveillance of health-care-associated infections (HAIs) can significantly improve the early detection of certain diseases, track the spread of illnesses, and generally help monitor and control the infections. In that way, successfully identifying "weak spots" to satisfy practitioners apply adequate preventive measures and act accordingly. An HAI surveillance program deploys databases derived from various sources to evaluate the emerging disease outbreaks to thoroughly analyze the patterns and indicators. In other words, an HAI program measures the incidence of HAIs and assesses the severity of diseases. In certain instances, it can help determine patient outcomes or measure the quality of care. Recent research suggests that HAI social networks of patients and caregivers, and data created from electronic health-care records (EHR) that are otherwise collected for other purposes, can successfully generate probabilistic simulations of nosocomial outbreaks of methicillin-resistant *Staphylococcus aureus* and influenza [13]. Similarly, electronic health records using machine learning applications have proven invaluable for predicting the risks of nosocomial *Clostridioides difficile* infection (CDI) [14], thus preventing or mitigating severe complications. The advantage of the machine learning approach to conventional CDI risk grouping is that the AI program refers to processing the existing risk factors and utilizes a wide range of variables within the EHR. Consequently, this technology can design different models to refer to the specific needs/activities of either patient or caregiver population. As the patient's CDI risk is likely to change over time during their inpatient stay, the machine learning application used for surveillance purposes is reported to act flawlessly and warn the caregivers of the unanticipated changes accordingly. Such a tailored approach to patients at high risks of developing CDI needs to be given further practical evidence in clinical trials and other relevant research studies that focus on HAI. However, it is apparent that it shows strong potential of upgrading HAI surveillance and IPC (infection prevention and control) and that similar or more advanced AI solutions would be considered invaluable.

Readiness to accurately discern CDI high-risk patients and timely respond with an appropriate intervention can integrate IPC and antimicrobial stewardship strategies and anti-CDI therapies [14]. Similarly, clinical trials of novel anti-SCI therapies and protocols developed for CDI high-risk patients could benefit from this approach.

AI data mining processes fulfill their purpose within the clinical microbiology lab to fulfill results, which could help uncover and forecast outbreaks of multidrug-resistant organism colonization and/or infection events. Observation of potential sources of the outbreaks, being generally considered a demanding segment of epidemiological investigation, could be accelerated by this kind of analysis. In that context, we witness more progressive use of the next-generation sequencing (NGS) for pathogen distinguishing, antimicrobial resistance (AMR) detection, and strain typing [15] as AI provides mechanisms for a more exhaustive analysis of NGS-generated information that would be created as an integrated segment of diverse HAI and AMR data merged from the available information collected throughout the health-care system. This could help track patients most at risk of HAI and AMR events, providing timely real-time insight into the interconnectedness of patients, clinics, and staff in molecular analysis of transmission events. Whereas our comprehension of cross-infection occurrence will thus be enhanced, other significant advances could also be made, such as timely diagnostic procedures and targeted IPC interventions.

On the other hand, certain major obstacles have been HAI surveillance reported for AI. It is a prerequisite that all the collected data should be of the highest quality to design precise and practically applicable models for each scenario/context. Recent research confirms that numerous studies in machine learning deal with too small datasets that they can neither grasp the potential nor evaluate the capability of AI programs and that a thorough authentication of predictions is necessary so that incorporation of findings into clinical practice is successfully implemented. What is more, as Fitzpatrick et al. (2020) observe, current databases might have been heavily biased by general clinical practice, which might affect the treatment once they become an integrative part of a machine learning model [16]. Another downside of AI in HAI might be the potential generalization of machine learning models for HAI surveillance which could not be applicable in every health-care setting. For instance, one CDI model can feature risk factors for CDI in one context, but they might not work in the same way for other settings [17].

7.4 The Applications of AI in the Novel Coronavirus (COVID-19) Outbreak

More recently, the implementation of the AI platform in the newly evolving coronavirus (COVID-19) environment has underlined its prospects of effective management of public health in unexpected disease outbreaks. In cases of immediate danger arising from sudden disease outbreaks, the AI concept can ensure the fast and secure decision- making process, given its capacity to analyze the vast amount of data inflow from various sources, such as government, social media, etc. AI-code identification may provide a more rapid contact identification across data and enable better assessment and optimization of IPC strategies to prevent cross-infection. Similarly, some platforms relative to air travel data incorporate machine learning, among other procedures, to process amounts of uncategorized data across various languages aiming at tracking outbreaks among no fewer than 100 diseases. BlueDot, one of these platforms, was used for the first time during the COVID-19 outbreak in December 2019, pinpointing the occurrence of the disease outbreak an entire week before both the WHO and national disease surveillance centers registered the phenomenon.

The crucial superiority of the application on global-scale outbreaks is the fact that it can also be applied locally within IPC teams, which implies that AI-generated data analytics may help public health professionals address programs that will focus on minimizing cross-infections instead of collecting data and writing up the reports.

- **Artificial Intelligence and Hand Hygiene**

The infection prevention and control (IPC) program has hand hygiene as one of the critical aspects. Technology in hand hygiene may offer to augment and adjust IPC procedures through novel guidance procedures and surveys. The SureWash system is commonly used as a widely accessible interactive booth with AR-powered surveillance to instruct and evaluate hygiene methods, gaining higher hygiene performance.

The very mobility of the booth facilitates its utilization by health-care staff, which can use it when needed, with immediate individual feedback on the quality of the hygiene performance.

It was only lately, the system was available through a smartphone application for similar purposes. "A pilot of an integrated hand hygiene digital framework that included the SureWash system and a hand hygiene auditing tool and an activity monitoring system demonstrated the feasibility of using AI without impairing clinical workflow" [18].

"Risk status" management was illustrated to the staff within a substantial number of formats, encompassing activities intended for increasing the score. AI application could also be extended to ensure that this dataset is supplemented with the HAI observation data that enables foreseeing possible outbreaks in the future and making recommendations of IPC interventions.

Computer vision deals with how humans perceive images and their content. In a virtual clinical ambiance, where persons are presented only as contours with no specific features, the AI system for monitoring hand hygiene detected more successfully hand alcohol dispersion than the subsequent hand rubbing [19]. As suggested by Lacey et al. (2020), the implementation of the real-time feedback for AI sensed a change in behavior patterns in specific situations had been attributed particular importance [20]. In their study of handwashing behavior recorded at clinical wards, sink surveillance was immensely helpful at improving both the quality and quantity of handwashing.

However, in the absence of the video monitoring system, earlier patterns of behavior were regained, which suggests that the application of the AI monitoring system is necessary as an infection prevention measure [20].

In their analysis of other issues concerning vision-based systems, Haque et al. observed that video surveillance system also involves some privacy issues (limiting the visual data that can be used, challenges around hospital infrastructure). There also remains the unresolved issue of how best to take account of people traffic in real life rather than in the quieter simulation setting [21].

Wearable technologies aimed at hygiene improvement in the health-care environment are given full attention. The potential for enhancing machine learning-based applications will positively ensure the maintenance of improved hygiene patterns of behavior among health-care staff. The study of sustainable improvements in maintaining hand hygiene monitored by video surveillance systems is far from being achieved. The behavior monitored varied greatly (between 6 and 54%), as suggested by Meng et al. (2019) [22].

In conclusion, the continuous wearing of the apparatus may seriously affect the user's attitude and hamper its functionality. For example, auditory or visual reminders to the user may affect their operation, especially those in palliative care.

Finally, the aspects that remain to be observed are the device design, size, or weight, as these may be perceived as "shackles" in providing care to patients. One of the viable solutions to this problem is the wrist wearable design of the system.

- **Artificial Intelligence and Oral Hygiene**

The goal of oral hygiene is to regularly eliminate plaque that forms around the gingival margin and proximal tooth surface in order to prevent oral colonization, which presents itself as a crucial element in causing caries. The use of a mouthwash, toothbrush, or a combination of the two, along with suctioning secretions, should be the norm when it comes to cleaning teeth. People's way of brushing teeth is constantly being enhanced as newer electric toothbrushes are released into the market. Accuracy, duration, and frequency are just some parameters that smart toothbrushes analyze. They have integrated 3D sensors that are capable of noticing position and orientation in different brushing fields in real time.

Now, behaviors regarding oral hygiene are traced by usual indicators. These indicators include dental plaque, periodontal inflammation, and caries, in addition to the patient being able to report their oral hygiene practices during a clinic visit. When major groups of people are involved, though, these tend to become exhausting; this is especially true if said people do not enjoy the privilege of regular access to dental services. The outcome, for example, plaque and dental disease, which is observed in-clinic visits, could be more thoroughly explained with the implementation of new systems that could show us the connection between oral hygiene behaviors and said outcome. Dental professionals are required to emphasize the importance of oral hygiene. This could be achieved by including real-time surveillance and feedback capacities which could then lead to better adherence of patients to oral practices. In addition, this would also show why people tend to or do not follow suggested oral hygiene practices. For quality patient-centered care to be provided, the use of smart systems in a mix with oral hygiene practice measurement and feedback devices is suggested, in addition to them being back-ended by risk prediction and customized prevention algorithms. This would give a digitally involved patient more control over their oral health and subsequently make them more involved.

The device can track skipped places and offer custom suggestions in regard to oral care, thanks to artificial intelligence (AI) and machine learning algorithms. User application of too much pressure and teeth that require more attention and percentage of brushed surface are all shown on a tooth map. Suppose the person applies too many pressure tests possible to cause gingival damage; therefore, it's important to prevent that. Thanks to AI-powered examinations, patients have no trouble getting a total and accurate mouth cleaning. This includes enhancing their technique, completion of brushing on missed surfaces, and maintaining not too harsh of a pressure. In no time, they will have a perfect oral hygiene routine without missing a tooth. Serious caries complications can be prevented by involving smart toothbrushes in a hygiene program. One issue that needs to be approached directly and further investigated for the implementation of these devices is their marginal markup in price in comparison to standard toothbrushes. They usually have a replaceable brush head but lack the ability to sterilize the fixed body.

7.5 Artificial Intelligence Algorithms and Nutrition in Preventive Dentistry

One of the most important segments of preventive dentistry is the observation of patient's nutritional habits. Many oral diseases, primarily caries, are directly linked with the type of food we eat and the individual's food intake frequency. Clinical nutrients research, which is being progressively conducted through advanced AI algorithms, finds its application in dietary activities support systems, food-related dental diseases risks, and general nutrient habits.

AI in dietary assessment mobile applications has found its significance in the field of prophylaxis. In a research study published in 2008, Sun et al. reported on a successful design of an electronic photographic method and associated image processing algorithms to approximate food intake [23]. In a more recent publication, Lu et al. (2020) offered goFOODTM as an artificial dietary evaluation system based on AI, requiring input information through sample photographs taken by a smartphone [23]. This simple system calculates the calorie and macronutrient content of a meal, thus providing a reliable dietary assessment. Similarly, Yang et al. (2019) suggested a new methodological approach in nutritional epidemiology, Ontology for Nutritional Epidemiology (ONE), as an authentic tool utilized for easier integration, visibility, and connectedness of research findings in the field of nutritional epidemiology [24]. The research showcases a more objective dietary assessment. A group of researchers (Lo et al. 2018) designed a dietary evaluation system based on a specific neural network to calculate food volume [25]. A set of visual data was utilized to develop a neural network by applying the deep learning approach. Mobile phone images of food portions were also the data input for another group of researchers [26], who approximated food energy based on images and the generative adversarial network (GAN) architecture over a time span a week with a sample of 45 respondents [26]. Another image-based research study [27] appraised the respective rationality of an image-based dietary evaluation app entitled Keenoa, designed through the food diary notes of a group of a hundred adults during a 3-day period [27]. The research showcased that the Keenoa app has demonstrated significant advantages if utilized for dietary assessment of the general population, whereas its use for personal assessment remains prone to errors. One similar research project [28] centered around the application of AI in nutrition deployed the fuzzy decision model for designing an online support system aiming to browse the available food constitution databases as a basis for calculating dietary intake [28]. The rationale behind this research project was the necessity of designing guidelines for Taiwanese dietary practitioners who are reported to have poor databases of Chinese menus and need a reliable decision-making tool.

As AI technology has obviously found its application assessing nutrition in terms of their quality and quantity, many research studies only confirmed that there might be room for designing AI apps and tools that deal with the amount of nutrients spent. The significance of these research findings could be best showcased in terms of the obesity epidemic the world has been facing at present. For instance, the Internet of Things (IoT) approach was deployed to develop a monitoring system that tracks personal activities through sensors on a smart-log patch, with the data later processed through a Bayesian deep learning network (EC-BDLN). Another study explored a similar approach to e-health applications related to cardio-metabolic caries risk factors in the general population [29, 30]. Ramyaa et al. (2019) investigated to what extent AI technology can assist in determining a set of observable traits in female built if machine studying, support vector machine (SVM), neural network, and k-nearest neighbor (kNN) calculations are deployed.

However, despite of the fact that the application of AI is more on nutrient studies, there is a considerable lack of more complex algorithms that could be utilized for similar purposes. Based on the available studies, it can be concluded that one of the under-research AI contexts might be inadequate or lacking incorporation with research on the use of medical robotics. One of the suggested solutions to this issue may be requirements to change the mindset and skills of practitioners, which is in line with the demands of future research in both medical and food industries [31].

7.6 AI and Prevention of Dental Trauma

Although dental injuries seen in toddlers and teenagers occur on a regular basis and are a common health situation to be dealt with by dental practitioners, the incidence of these occurrences has increased in the last two decades. As per rule, dental injuries are always regarded as an emergency, and they require instant action to help lessen the pain and treat teeth displacement or injured tissue. Adequate diagnostic procedures and dental practitioner's timely reactions can guarantee successful recovery. Clinical practice confirms that the more thorough the examination, the more successful the treatment. In addition to this, the proper reaction and detailed examination along with skills in traumatology can help patients overcome anxiety or stress and ease the dental team operations. A practical application system of AI is known as knowledge-based systems (KBS). This system provides significant assistance to caregivers.

With the helping hand of AI, a widely known program (XpertRule, Attar, London) can be used to cross-analyze the input data and predict dental injuries with children. With the context given, such information can be further deployed to prevent dental trauma or provide a summary of children's behavior patterns when active. The prevention can be enhanced by using mouth guards and helmets during sports activities.

7.7 AI in Periodontal Risk Assessment

Periodontitis appears to be one of the most common dental diseases in the general adult population. Every second a person over 50 years of age suffers from this disease and thus is likely to become toothless during their lifetimes. According to the definition, periodontitis starts as a severe gum infection. Still, it develops in a complex inflammatory disease that damages soft tissues, both the tissues anchoring the tooth root in its bone and the gingiva. When the disease progresses, it causes the increase of gingival crevices and the development of periodontal pockets, leading to loss of teeth [32]. In order to prevent complications, AI technology is believed to introduce solutions that might help cure this largely preventable disease. An innovative machine-based learning analysis that included numerous medical and sociodemographic features of the general population showcased that periodontitis, like any chronic condition typical of an older population, bears linkage to a structural risk pattern contrary to belief not rooted in poor oral habits or other relevant stressors. As the database did not contain oral hygiene-related variables such as plaque index, which can make a difference between gingival inflammations caused by gingival inflammation and those not related to oral hygiene, the structural risk pattern could not be predicted at all [33]. The chosen variables included by the algorithm were generally known risk factors such as smoking, female hormones, or age.

The machine learning approach provides a risk score for periodontitis based on personalized characteristics, excluding local factors. AI technology can easily recognize individuals that are likely to develop periodontitis, provided a compound range of variables are deployed, including medical, sociodemographic, or genetic factors. If the machine learning findings are utilized as complementary data that support diagnostics of risk-prone patients, preventive measures may be better tailored to achieve success.

7.8 Artificial Intelligence and Caries Prevention

Dental caries or tooth decay is a common transmissible disease influenced by a combination of various environmental and genetic factors. Even though advanced tools for evaluating caries risks have been developed, no studies showcase models designed to predict caries risks that refer to new factors (i.e., human genetic factors). As recent research suggests, the most frequent chronic disease in 2016 across the globe was teeth caries. Globally, the treatment of caries skyrocketed in 2015, reaching 540 billion dollars, thus overburdening dental clinics [34]. These statistics call for immediate measures in preventing caries risks.

Research studies have demonstrated shift in the distribution of caries, as it was mainly adolescents who were reported to be suffering from this disease in the general population [35]. Recommendations of scholars who participated in the conference of National Institutes of Health Consensus Development (2001) aimed at emphasizing that much attention should be paid to individuals that are risk-prone to help prevent and control dental caries. As caries can be successfully prevented, the utilization of AI-based tools and applications for implementing risk prediction models in early diagnostics and precise examinations in adolescents likely to develop caries would be considered highly beneficial.

Caries risk predicting models (CRPMs) are reported to be significantly successful in the improvement of patient's care due to their being noninvasive treatment approaches. These models feature general flexibility to permit patients to decide on how deceptive intervention they choose [36]. In that context, it is currently adopted that four standardized caries risk evaluation models are generally used: ADA (American Dental Association), CAT (Caries-Risk Assessment Tool), CAMBRA (Caries Management by Risk Assessment), and Cariogram. All four models deal with the same variables that refer only to environmental indicators and behavioral factors, including plaque index, the number of *Streptococcus mutans* and *Lactobacillus*, saliva flow, and salivary buffer capacity. There is a consensus that the Cariogram seems to be the one more advance and accurate of all the mentioned CRPMs for certain tests. However, it fails to prove its efficiency in caries prediction. As evidenced in Cagetti et al. (2018), Cariogram demonstrates different sensitivity scopes, ranging from 41.0 to 75.0%, whereas the specificity ranged from 65.8 to 88.0% [36].

What causes and develops dental caries is a systemic interconnection of genetic and environmental risk factors. As for the caries risk factors related to the environment, it is reported that dietary exposure to sugar, poor hygiene habits, features and flow of saliva, and dental plaque are the most common determining factors [37]. On the other hand, factors stemming from genetics also have a high ratio of impact, as it is reported that the genetic risk score variation is 49.1–62.7% [38]. Caries risk, being a specific genetical phenotype, is affected by various other factors that can contribute to individual conditions. Along with the genetic factors, there are additional variables that relate to food consumption habits, immune system quality, saliva characteristics, taste, or enamel formation [39]. The latter factor, as a group of scholars found, adds to caries development risks, as a relationship between enamelin (ENAM) and high risk of caries. In addition to this, research studies confirm that "a relationship between the genetic variation of tuftelin (TUFT1) and caries could be observed only when the Streptococcus mutans levels were high" [40]. In that context, relying on CRPMs environmental-based factors only risks losing much useful information. Some research studies propose that if a combined risk prediction model consisting of both genetic and environmental factors is designed and utilized, it provides a more precise prediction in tracking either of these two factors than when used solely.

This implies that CRPMs need to be explored and researched with practical implications related to both groups of factors so that predicting caries risk could be conducted with more accuracy. A CRPM showcased in the study of Geilleit et al. (2018) is an innovative caries risk prediction model that is the first one to be designed with both mentioned predictors. By utilizing ML algorithms, this model includes, among others, factors such as "cariostatic score," "plaque index," and "past caries experience," the latter of which appeared to be one of the most significant predictors of individual risk. Interestingly, this CRPM model included a factor that confirms whether the patients "were only teenagers in the family" [41].

In a similar Cariogram model developed by Ramesh et al. (2013), instead of "bacterial counts," "cariostatic score" was utilized for assessment of the cariogenic ability of the dental plaque. Cariostat, in fact deploys "a colorimetric test to evaluate the acid produced by bacteria in the plaque" [42]. As demonstrated in Richards et al.'s (2017) research study, carious lesions' development occurs due to bacterial acids affecting the dental tissues causing their demineralization [43]. The demineralization process is triggered when the pH level on teeth surfaces drops to <5.5. In that sense, Cariostat as a model can successfully evaluate the microbiological quality of caries and, quite contrary to other cariogenic tests such as Dentocult SM, focuses on the bacteria assessment and not the saliva in plaque. This model promises to provide more precision in the evaluation as cariogenic bacteria develop in the plaque form. Overall, as these studies imply that CRPM models provide substantial informational support, legislators could bring more informed decisions on prevention policies for high-risk groups in the general population.

With nearly 1.8 billion new cases every year across the globe, early globally, early childhood caries (ECC) have chronic childhood disease. To improve early childhood caries (ECC) detection and implement novel treatment strategies, AI can offer innovative and reliable solutions, mainly if combined with interactive oral health education delivered through smartphone applications. The main reason biomedical techniques in ECC control that are used presently have poor results is the fact that they mainly deal with individual cases in terms of treatment procedures and do not focus on the preventive aspects that would refer to the general population. In the early stages of caries development, when white lesions appear on the enamel surface, dental caries must be localized in order to prevent further tooth decay and its impact on dental hard tissues.

7.9 AI in Detection of Early Childhood Caries

The disease of early childhood caries (ECC) has been the most significant health problem and an international health challenge for children and their caregivers across the globe.

It is reported that the disease develops as a complex condition influenced by poor health hygiene, unbalanced diet, bacteria, and other determining risk factors [44]. To tackle the issue, parents and dental practitioners must act accordingly to diminish the risk factors and decrease the disease occurrence by self-engagement. As one of the key factors to overcome the problem is the caregiver's ignorance or poor knowledge of the possible emergence of this condition, it is necessary to develop strategies that deploy innovative artificial intelligence (AI)-powered smartphone applications, as they can be easily navigated by children or parents, especially if direct access to dental clinics is limited. Such a tool can additionally help raise awareness of the gravity of the problem and engage parents to reduce the caries risk in a more practical manner.

There is evidence that "managing individual behaviors conditions" by a smartphone application can result in positive outcomes such as weight loss, diminishing smoking habits, or Parkinson's disease progression [45, 46]. Statistics confirm that a significant percentage of Americans in the general population nowadays possess a smartphone (77%). In contrast, there is 85% of those coming from poorer backgrounds have access to smartphones [47]. This implies that, with such a high ratio of smartphone users, changes can be introduced in oral health interventions, making them more approachable and fun at the same time.

In the context of AI in dentistry, mobile dentistry as a growing scientific field has been introduced in academic communities to bring oral health issues to a broader focus of the general population. Unfortunately, the existing apps have certain limitations and cannot reach wider audiences. Firstly, the number of available apps for oral hygiene is significantly smaller than those that deal with general health issues. Secondly, of those applications that are commercially available, the majority focuses on the practical aspects of dental hygiene or recognition of specific dental diseases. The market has not yet offered a solution to communicate directly with parents and provide AI support for early caries detection in children. This is surprising, especially if we consider that AI image technology has been successfully utilized to support many disease diagnoses in various fields such as oncology, ophthalmology, radiology, etc. [48]. Smartphone applications (AICaries), specifically designed for parents-users, allow taking high- precision photos of their children's teeth. Thus, upon detection of ECC, children's caregivers can contact dental practitioners for initial treatment. In addition to this, such a smart app can serve as a training tool for parents who need further education on preventing ECC and eventually reducing caries risks.

References

1. Topol EJ (2019) High-performance medicine: the convergence of human and artificial intelligence. Nat Med 25(1):44–56. https://doi.org/10.1038/s41591-018-0300-7
2. Schwalbe N, Wahl B (2020) Artificial intelligence and the future of global health. Lancet 395(10236):1579–1586. https://doi.org/10.1016/s0140-6736(20)30226-9
3. Hosny A, Aerts H (2019) Artificial intelligence for global health. Science 366(6468):955–956. https://doi.org/10.1126/science.aay5189
4. Gyawali B (2018) Does global oncology need artificial intelligence? Lancet Oncol 19(5):599–600. https://doi.org/10.1016/s1470-2045(18)30269-9
5. Mishra SR, Neupane D, Preen D, Kallestrup P, Perry HB (2015) Mitigation of non-communicable diseases in developing countries with community health workers. Glob Health 11(1):43. https://doi.org/10.1186/s12992-015-0129-5
6. Susskind RSD (2016) Technology will replace many doctors, lawyers, and other professionals. Harvard Business Review [cited 2016 Oct 16]. Available from: https://hbr.org/2016/10/robots-will-replace-doctors- lawyers-and-other-professionals
7. Clarkson JE, Ramsay CR, Eccles MP, Eldridge S, Grimshaw JM, Johnston M et al (2010) The translation research in a dental setting (TRiaDS) programme protocol. Implement Sci 5(1):57. https://doi.org/10.1186/1748-5908-5-57
8. Sahrish T, Nidhi G, Preety G, Aditi S (2021) Artificial intelligence in public health dentistry. *Inter Healthcare Res J 5*(9):RV1–RV5. https://doi.org/10.26440/ihrj/0509.12489
9. Gupta S. The future of artificial intelligence in dentistry. Healthcare in America. 2020. August 20, 2018. Accessed 15 May 2020. https://healthcareinamerica.us/the-future-of-artificial-intelligence-in-dentistry- 114e04fc4e8f
10. Lavrac N (1999) Selected techniques for data mining in medicine. Artif Intell Med 16(1):3–23. https://doi.org/10.1016/s0933-3657(98)00062-1
11. Pretty IA, Maupomé G (2004) A closer look at diagnosis in clinical dental practice: part 3. Effectiveness of radiographic diagnostic procedures. J Can Dent Assoc 70(6):388–394
12. Balaban C (2021) Linda V. AI-Driven transformation of dental benefits. Compendium 42(6)
13. Cusumano-Towner M, Li DY, Tuo S, Krishnan G, Maslove DM (2013) A social network of hospital acquired infection built from electronic medical record data. J Am Med Informat Associat: JAMIA 20(3):427–434. https://doi.org/10.1136/amiajnl-2012-001401
14. Li BY, Oh J, Young VB, Rao K, Wiens J (2019) Using machine learning and the electronic health record to predict complicated Clostridium difficile infection. *Open Forum Infect Dis 6*(5):ofz186. https://doi.org/10.1093/ofid/ofz186
15. Deurenberg RH, Bathoorn E, Chlebowicz MA, Couto N, Ferdous M, García-Cobos S, Rossen JW (2017) Application of next generation sequencing in clinical microbiology and infection prevention. J Biotechnol 243:16–24. https://doi.org/10.1016/j.jbiotec.2016.12.022
16. Fitzpatrick F, Doherty A, Lacey G (2020) Using artificial intelligence in infection prevention. Curr Treat Options Infect Dis 12(2):135–144. https://doi.org/10.1007/s40506-020-00216-7
17. Oh J, Makar M, Fusco C, McCaffrey R, Rao K, Ryan EE et al (2018) A generalizable, data-driven approach to predict daily risk of clostridium difficile infection at two large academic health centers. Infect Control Hosp Epidemiol 39(4):425–433. https://doi.org/10.1017/ice.2018.16
18. Thirkell G, Chambers J, Gilbart W, Thornhill K, Arbogast J, Lacey G (2018) Pilot study of digital tools to support multimodal hand hygiene in a clinical setting. Am J Infect Control 46(3):261–265. https://doi.org/10.1016/j.ajic.2017.08.042
19. Awwad S, Tarvade S, Piccardi M, Gattas DJ (2019) The use of privacy-protected computer vision to measure the quality of healthcare worker hand hygiene. Int J Qual Health Care 31(1):36–42. https://doi.org/10.1093/intqhc/mzy099
20. Lacey G, Zhou J, Li X, Craven C, Gush C (2020) The impact of automatic video auditing with real- time feedback on the quality and quantity of handwash events in a hospital setting. Am J Infect Control 48(2):162–166. https://doi.org/10.1016/j.ajic.2019.06.015

21. Haque A, Guo M, Alahi A, Yeung S, Luo Z, Rege A, Fei-Fei L (2017) Towards vision-based smart hospitals: A system for tracking and monitoring hand hygiene compliance. In: Paper presented at the proceedings of the 2nd machine learning for healthcare conference. Research, Proceedings of Machine Learning. https://proceedings.mlr.press/v68/haque17a.html
22. Meng M, Sorber M, Herzog A, Igel C, Kugler C (2019) Technological innovations in infection control: A rapid review of the acceptance of behavior monitoring systems and their contribution to the improvement of hand hygiene. Am J Infect Control 47(4):439–447. https://doi.org/10.1016/j.ajic.2018.10.012
23. Sun M, Liu Q, Schmidt K, Yang J, Yao N, Fernstrom JD, Sclabassi RJ (2008) Determination of food portion size by image processing. Annu Int Conf IEEE Eng Med Biol Soc 2008:871–874. https://doi.org/10.1109/iembs.2008.4649292
24. Yang C, Ambayo H, Baets BD, Kolsteren P, Thanintorn N, Hawwash D et al (2019) An ontology to standardize research output of nutritional epidemiology: from paper-based standards to linked content. Nutrients 11(6):1300. https://doi.org/10.3390/nu11061300
25. Lo FPW, Sun Y, Qiu J, Lo B (2018) Food volume estimation based on deep learning view synthesis from a single depth map. Nutrients 10(12):2005. https://doi.org/10.3390/nu10122005
26. Fang S, Shao Z, Kerr DA, Boushey CJ, Zhu F (2019) An end-to-end image-based automatic food energy estimation technique based on learned energy distribution images: protocol and methodology. Nutrients 11(4). https://doi.org/10.3390/nu11040877
27. Ji Y, Plourde H, Bouzo V, Kilgour RD, Cohen TR (2020) Validity and usability of a smartphone image-based dietary assessment app compared to 3-day food diaries in assessing dietary intake among Canadian adults: randomized controlled trial. JMIR Mhealth Uhealth 8(9):e16953. https://doi.org/10.2196/16953
28. Hsu CY, Huang LC, Chen TM, Chen LF, Chao JC (2011) A web-based decision support system for dietary analysis and recommendations. Telemed J E Health 17(2):68–75. https://doi.org/10.1089/tmj.2010.0104
29. Ramyaa R, Hosseini O, Krishnan GP, Krishnan S (2019) Phenotyping women based on dietary macronutrients, physical activity, and body weight using machine learning tools. Nutrients 11(7). https://doi.org/10.3390/nu11071681
30. Tragomalou A, Moschonis G, Manios Y, Kassari P, Ioakimidis I, Diou C et al (2020) Novel e-health applications for the Management of Cardiometabolic Risk Factors in children and adolescents in Greece. Nutrients 12(5):1380
31. Akyazi T, Goti A, Oyarbide A, Alberdi E, Bayon F (2020) A guide for the food industry to meet the future skills requirements emerging with industry 4.0. *Foods 9*(4):492
32. Eke PI, Borgnakke WS, Genco RJ (2020) Recent epidemiologic trends in periodontitis in the USA. Periodontol 82(1):257–267. https://doi.org/10.1111/prd.12323
33. Bartold PM, Van Dyke TE (2017) Host modulation: controlling the inflammation to control the infection. Periodontol 75(1):317–329. https://doi.org/10.1111/prd.12169
34. Righolt AJ, Jevdjevic M, Marcenes W, Listl S (2018) Global-, regional-, and country-level economic impacts of dental diseases in 2015. J Dent Res 97(5):501–507. https://doi.org/10.1177/0022034517750572
35. Kaste LM, Selwitz RH, Oldakowski RJ, Brunelle JA, Winn DM, Brown LJ (1996) Coronal caries in the primary and permanent dentition of children and adolescents 1-17 years of age: United States, 1988-1991. J Dent Res 75:631–641. https://doi.org/10.1177/002203459607502s03
36. Doméjean S, Banerjee A, Featherstone JDB (2017) Caries risk/susceptibility assessment: its value in minimum intervention oral healthcare. Br Dent J 223(3):191–197. https://doi.org/10.1038/sj.bdj.2017.665
37. Selwitz RH, Ismail AI, Pitts NB (2007) Dental caries. Lancet 369(9555):51–59. https://doi.org/10.1016/s0140-6736(07)60031-2
38. Haworth S, Esberg A, Lif Holgerson P, Kuja-Halkola R, Timpson NJ, Magnusson PKE et al (2020) Heritability of caries scores, trajectories, and disease subtypes. J Dent Res 99(3):264–270. https://doi.org/10.1177/0022034519897910

39. Vieira AR, Modesto A, Marazita ML (2014) Caries: review of human genetics research. Caries Res 48(5):491–506. https://doi.org/10.1159/000358333
40. Slayton RL, Cooper ME, Marazita ML (2005) Tuftelin, mutans streptococci, and dental caries susceptibility. J Dent Res 84:711–714
41. Geilleit R, Hen ZQ, Chong CY, Loh AP, Pang NL, Peterson GM et al (2018) Feasibility of a real-time hand hygiene notification machine learning system in outpatient clinics. J Hosp Infect 100(2):183–189. https://doi.org/10.1016/j.jhin.2018.04.004
42. Ramesh K, Kunjappan S, Ramesh M, Shankar S, Reddy S (2013) Comparative evaluation of predictive value of three caries activity tests-Snyder, lactobacillus count and cariostat in mixed dentition children with and without caries. J Pharm Bioallied Sci 5(Suppl 1):S63–S68. https://doi.org/10.4103/0975-7406.113299
43. Richards VP, Alvarez AJ, Luce AR, Bedenbaugh M, Mitchell ML, Burne RA, Nascimento MM (2017) Microbiomes of site-specific dental plaques from children with different caries status. Infect Immun 85(8). https://doi.org/10.1128/iai.00106-17
44. Wu TT, Xiao J, Sohn MB, Fiscella KA, Gilbert C, Grier A et al (2021) Machine learning approach identified multi-platform factors for caries prediction in child-mother dyads. Front Cell Infect Microbiol 11:727630. https://doi.org/10.3389/fcimb.2021.727630
45. Ernsting C, Dombrowski SU, Oedekoven M, Kanzler M, Kuhlmey A, Gellert P (2017) Using smartphones and health apps to change and manage health behaviors: A population-based survey. J Med Internet Res 19(4):e101. https://doi.org/10.2196/jmir.6838
46. Wang J, Wang Y, Wei C, Yao NA, Yuan A, Shan Y, Yuan C (2014) Smartphone interventions for long-term health management of chronic diseases: an integrative review. Telemed J E Health 20(6):570–583. https://doi.org/10.1089/tmj.2013.0243
47. Chowdhry A. Lower-income Americans are becoming increasingly dependent on smartphones, says study. Forbes. 2018 March 13. URL: https://www.forbes.com/sites/amitchowdhry/2017/03/13/lower-income- americans-are-becoming-increasingly-dependent-on-smartphones-says-study/?sh=644075941083
48. Xiao J, Luo J, Ly-Mapes O, Wu TT, Dye T, Al Jallad N et al (2021) Assessing a smartphone app (AICaries) that uses artificial intelligence to detect dental caries in children and provides interactive Oral health education: protocol for a design and usability testing study. JMIR Res Protoc 10(10):e32921. https://doi.org/10.2196/32921

Chapter 8
Artificial Intelligence-Based Dental Diseases Through X-Ray Images Using Entropy CNN-Based and Support Fusion Mating

8.1 Introduction

Dental caries is a chronic infectious oral disease that affects the majority of teenagers and adults around the world. According to the National Health and Nutrition Examination Survey, dental caries affects 41% of children aged 2–11 years (in their primary teeth), 42% of children and adolescents aged 6–19 years, and 90% of people aged 20 years (in their permanent teeth). The majority of research has found that socially and economically disadvantaged people, such as low-income minorities, those with lower levels of education, and people with disabilities, are more likely to develop dental caries [1]. Dental caries afflicted 621 million children globally in 2017 [2]. With a 20.6% increase over a decade [3], the prevalence of permanent dental caries among 12-year-olds in China increased by 7.8% between 2007 and 2017 [4]. Age, sex, social determinants (income and education), health-related habits (smoking, food, alcohol consumption, and health-care attendance), and water fluoridation all play a role in dental caries [5].

Furthermore, various epidemiological and clinical research have shown that tooth loss caused by oral illness, such as dental caries, is linked to negative dietary changes as well as potentially modifiable risk factors or risk indicators for cardiovascular disease and cognitive impairment. Various retention and restoration strategies for the treatment of dental cavities have been proposed and improved over the last few decades [6]. With the rapid advancement of technology, image processing techniques have seen tremendous success and appeal in a wide range of applications. Alternatively, dental caries is regarded as the most widespread and quickly spreading disease. The bacteria (found in plaque) break down the food in the teeth, generating acids that severely damage the hard tissues around the teeth, resulting in tooth decay or dental caries. Approximately 60–90 percent of schoolchildren are impacted by this widely distributed disease, which is still considered a serious health problem. Recently, image processing techniques have been used in dentistry

K. Shaikh et al., *Artificial Intelligence in Dentistry*,
https://doi.org/10.1007/978-3-031-19715-4_8

to aid in the early detection and diagnosis of dental caries and other oral illnesses. It simply defines and categorizes the many types of dental disease infections. Several studies have been conducted for the detection of dental caries in difficult situations, and multiple approaches for the classification of dental caries are advised. Nonetheless, no such system can accurately characterize caries layers. However, in recent years, several ML (machine learning) techniques have been used to identify and analyze image data. The ANN (artificial neural network) and DNN (deep neural network) models of the ML method stand out among them. Despite the multiple existing strategies for early caries diagnosis, it is critical to develop a precise caries detection technique that is advantageous to the dentist [7].

In clinical orthodontic diagnosis, dental models play a significant role. By extracting, moving, and rearranging the teeth from the dental models, they can truly demonstrate the 3D anatomy structure of patients with malocclusion, as well as the form and position distribution of the teeth, and assist dentists in designing an effective and precise dental treatment plan. As a result, tooth segmentation is an essential stage in many oral medical research processes, as well as the foundation for computer-assisted dental diagnosis and therapy [8]. Gingivitis is an inflammation of the gingiva all-around tooth that causes the gums to become sensitive and bleed. Gingivitis can proceed to periodontitis, which causes severe inflammation and infection in the teeth's supporting tissues. Due to soft tissue inflammation and bone loss, periodontal disease is a leading cause of tooth loss in adults. Periodontal disease has been shown as a significant predictor of oral-systemic health [9].

The fissures in the occlusal surface of the tooth are often where dental caries begin. Visual inspection, tactile sense, and radiography are the mainstays of traditional caries examinations [10]. A panoramic radiograph is one of the most common dental radiographic examinations because it allows for the screening of a large anatomical region while only using a little amount of radiation. Although panoramic radiographs have not previously been considered for tooth recognition and numbering, similar approaches have been investigated for other forms of radiographs such as medical computed tomography (CT) and bitewings [11]. As assumed, most individuals have 32 teeth in total (eight teeth on each side of the jaw), which means we have 32 dental positions to detect. Meanwhile, the medical x-ray image is poor due to patient privacy concerns, and we rarely have access to as much x-ray picture data as we would like. As a result, tooth recognition and classification based on a high number of classes vs. a small amount of visual data is difficult. Many researchers have used image processing and segmentation techniques to achieve automatic tooth recognition using x-ray image preprocessing and teeth segmentation [12]. Furthermore, some patients may be wearing dental accessories at the time of the radiology. Such foreign objects disrupt the feature distribution of each tooth, making the segmentation job more difficult. Traditional geometry-based approaches are less suitable for teeth segmentation tasks in practice as a result of these limitations, as they are less robust to complicated tooth forms and tooth configurations [13].

Observers have major disagreements over whether caries lesions are visible even when using the same radiograph. The quality of the radiograph, how the dentist views it and the time it takes to perform each exam can all affect inter-rater agreement. When 34 raters viewed the same bitewing radiographs in a previous study, the mean kappa values for the presence or absence of dental caries and their degree ranged from 0.30 to 0.72. Consistency is crucial, especially when it comes to detecting the early stages of dental caries [14]. Deep learning and convolutional neural networks (CNNs) have lately been actively researched for the interpretation of various types of medical pictures, with encouraging findings [15].

The following is how the paper is organized: The associated works are discussed in Sect. 8.2. The proposed methodology is explained in Sect. 8.3, and the findings and debate are covered in Sect. 8.4. The conclusion is followed by the reference section in Sect. 8.5.

8.2 Related Works

Various strategies for computer-aided image segmentation in dentistry have been reported in the literature [16, 17]. This study tried to evaluate whether VRF could be recognized using panoramic radiography and convolutional neural network (CNN) technology, as employed by Fukuda et al. [18]. In this procedure, 330 VRF teeth with clearly visible fracture lines were selected from 330 panoramic photos in the hospital imaging collection. The presence of VRF lines was confirmed by two radiologists and an endodontist. A total of 240 photographs were assigned to a training set and 60 images to a test set out of the 300 total. To detect VRFs, DIGITS version 5.01 was used to develop CNN-based deep learning models. The precision of the implemented method was 0.93, and the F-measure was 0.83. Even though many studies have been published on the recognition of objects of interest from dental X-ray pictures, there is still a need for an automated technique that can accurately and effectively detect the required objects.

Xuan Zhang et al. [19] introduced a deep learning method based on a convolutional neural network (ConvNet) to detect dental caries from oral photos. For the construction and evaluation of the model, researchers used 3932 oral photos taken by 625 volunteers with consumer cameras. Adapting from Single Shot MultiBox Detector, a deep ConvNet was created. The model was automatically trained using the hard negative mining technique. The model was tested for (i) classification accuracy in detecting dental caries in photographs and (ii) localization accuracy in predicting the locations of anticipated dental caries. The deep learning model appears to be capable of detecting dental cavities in oral images taken with consumer cameras. It has the potential to aid in the early and cost-effective detection of dental caries in huge populations.

In-Ae Kang et al. [20] presented their findings. Dental caries is an infectious condition that causes tooth decay, with cavities being the most prevalent symptom. Dental caries are one of the most common oral health problems, and research has been conducted to improve early identification due to pain and treatment costs. Artificial intelligence has been used in recent years to develop models that can predict the risk of dental caries. Medical research in oral health care has shown limitations such as significant funds and time required; therefore, artificial intelligence has been used in recent years to develop models that can predict the risk of dental caries. The data for this study came from a survey of children's dental health done by the Korean Center for Disease Control and Prevention in 2018. The accuracy, F1-score, precision, and recall of several machine learning methods were used to evaluate their performance on this data. With an accuracy of 92 percent, an F1 score of 90 percent, a precision of 94 percent, and a recall of 87 percent, random forest has outperformed all other machine learning algorithms.

Rodolfo Reda et al. [21] addressed the existing evidence supporting the use of magnetic resonance imaging (MRI), a nonionizing radiation-free diagnostic scan, in several dental domains. Background: In today's first- and second-level dental diagnoses and treatment planning, radiographic imaging plays a critical role. The biggest downside is that patients are exposed to a lot of ionizing radiation. Methods: The PubMed electronic database was used to search for literature on dental MRI, and 37 research were found. Only the most relevant articles in the fields of endodontics, conservative dentistry, implantology, and oral and craniofacial surgery were chosen. The findings of all of the articles included in this review demonstrated that MRI can produce well-defined pictures that can be used in surgical dentistry. Conclusions: The promise of MRI for diagnosis in dental clinical practice is highlighted in this review, with minimal danger of biological damage from constant ionizing radiation exposure.

8.3 Proposed Methodology

The dental imaging collection, which was obtained from Noor Medical Imaging Center in Qom, Iran, consists of unidentified and anonymized panoramic dental x-ray images of 116 patients. From healthy teeth to partial and total edentulous instances, this dataset covers a wide range of dental disorders. Two dentists manually segment all conditions of distinct situations [14]. The dataset can be obtained from the Kaggle website which is publicly available at https:// www.kaggle.com/daverattan/dental-xrary-tfrecords.

8.3.1 Preprocessing

The multiclass classification will be performed using x-ray pictures of teeth in this study. There are three categories in this classification: "cavity," "filling," and "implant." The suggested effort will enrich the data at the beginning and then preprocess it. The data is then divided into training and validation sets. Consider ΔD is the x-ray image database, $\Delta D \in \{D1, D2, D3, ... Dn\}$, where "$n$" is the number of images and the vector function. For noise removal, the input images are first preprocessed with a Gaussian filtering function. A linear filter is a Gaussian filter. Where the underlying goal is to estimate the original image by suppressing noise from a noise-contaminated version of the image, filters are employed to increase. Equation [22] defines the Gaussian filter (8.1):

$$G_D(p,q) = \frac{1}{2\pi\delta_D^{\ 2}} \exp\frac{\left(-a^2 + b^2\right)}{2\delta_D^{\ 2}} \tag{8.1}$$

where (a, b) is the current pixel of the image. Figure 8.1 shows the proposed flowchart.

8.3.1.1 Convolution Entropy-Based Feature Mapping

CNN can extract powerful features from input data by building several filters and using these filters to extract representative features layer by layer. There are three types of layers in the current CNN feature extraction stage. The neural network in modified entropy-based convolution has four layers, plus one extra layer to normalize the structure, as shown in Fig. 8.2.

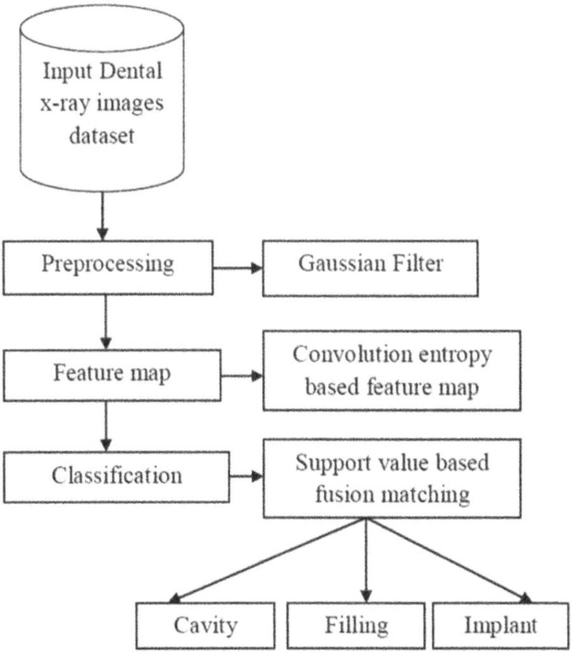

Fig. 8.1 The proposed flow diagram

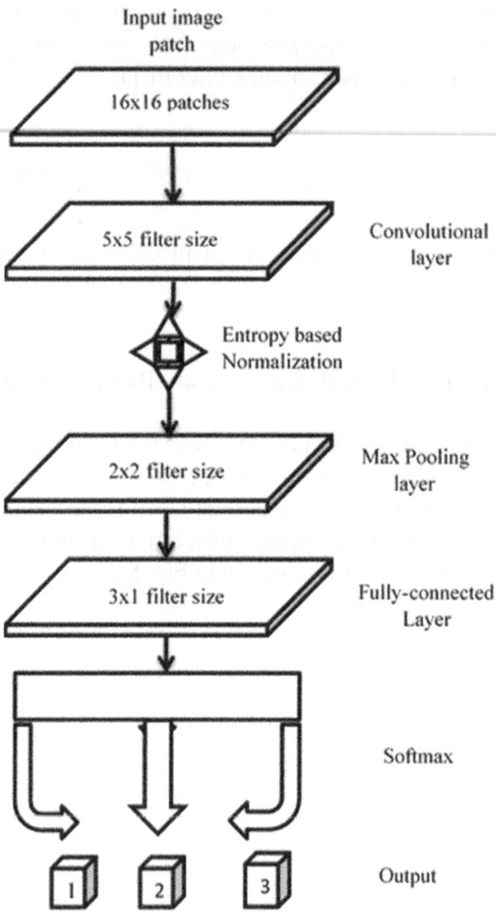

Fig. 8.2 The structure of a convolutional neural network

Convolutional Layer

It consists of numerous learned weight matrices (filters) that slide across the input characteristics. The yield of previous layers is convolved with distinct learning weight matrices called filter masks in each convolutional layer. The result is then prepared using a nonlinear procedure to create the layer output. Using conditional logic, this layer performs the convolution of the input data with the kernel (8.1). The result of the convolution is also known as the feature map:

$$C_k = \sum_{m=0}^{M-1} \Delta W_l y_n \hat{h}_{k-n} + \Delta B_n \tag{8.2}$$

where y_n is the input features, $\hat{h}$ is a filter, and M is the number of components in y and the output vector is C_k. The weights and biases of the model are updated with condition (8.3) and condition (8.4) separately for all layers:

$$\Delta W_l = -\frac{x\lambda}{r} W_n - \frac{x}{N_t} \frac{\partial C}{\partial W_n} + m\Delta W_n(t) \tag{8.3}$$

$$\Delta B_n = -\frac{x}{n} \frac{\partial C}{\partial B_n} + m\Delta B_n(t) \tag{8.4}$$

where W_n denotes the weight, B_n denotes the bias, n denotes the layer number, λ denotes the regularization parameter, x denotes the learning rate, N_t denotes the total number of training samples, m denotes the momentum, t denotes the updating step, and C denotes the cost function.

Entropy-Based Normalization Layer Feature Mapping

The output of the convolution layer is subjected to an entropy-based normalizing layer. The entropy-based normalization in the neural network is used to reduce overfitting in the layers before the max-pooling layer. Enthalpy is a haphazardness assessment that is used to describe the texture of an input image. This entropy value is used to distinguish between the texture of an iris and non-iris parts such as the sclera and pupil. The entropy of the ith superpixel E_y^i is calculated by condition (8.5) as

$$E_y^i = \sum_{u=0}^{m-1}\sum_{v=0}^{m-1} C_k(u,v)\left(-\log_2\left(C_k(u,v)\right)\right) \tag{8.5}$$

where u, v is the position value of C_k. The entropy of segmented contour-based features such as color, texture, and brightness is examined here, and the entropy features set is used as an input to the normalization procedure for effective clustering of the sclera, iris, and pupil segments separately.

(a) **Normalization**

Normalization is the process of linearly transforming data to fit it into a specific range. The enthalpy value determines the specific range in this case. For data standardization, the Z-score normalization is used, which linearly changes the data.

Equation (8.5) is the formula for Z-score normalization:

$$Z_{norm} = \frac{E_y^i - \mu}{\sigma} \tag{8.6}$$

Here, Z_{norm} is the normalized output, E_y^i is the entropy value, μ is the mean value of the convolutional layer output image, andσ is the standard deviation of the values in the convolutional layer output image. The entropy measure is used to normalize the output image of the convolutional layer (8.5). The entropy-based normalized image produced by this layer is fed into the pooling layer.

Pooling Layer

The downsampling layer is what it's called. To reduce the computational intensity and avoid overfitting, the pooling mechanism reduces the dimension of result neurons from the entropy-based normalization layer. The most extreme incentive in each element is chosen by max-pooling activity, which reduces the number of output neurons. Furthermore, the pooling layers help to simplify the data in the convolutional layer's output.

Fully Connected Layer

Each activation in the previous layer is fully associated with this layer. That is, each neuron from the maximum pooled layer is connected to all of the output neurons through this layer. The activation function used in this research is as follows:

Softmax
The probability distribution of the k output classes is calculated using this activation function. As a result, the output layer employs the softmax function to forecast a class input that fits the terms "cavity," "filling," and "implant":

$$p_i = \frac{e^{x_i}}{\sum_1^k e^{x_i}} \tag{8.7}$$

where x is the system input. Output feature mapping of CNN are "cavity," "filling," and "implant" segments. Convolutional neural networks have less difficulty to train convolution layers that are used to group images, feature map them by similarity, and conduct x-ray image identification in scenes.

8.3.2 *Classification of Support Value-Based Fusion Matching Process*

In this part, a support value-based fusion matching technique is used to match recognized and non-recognized proficient validation information. First, the support esteem for the extracted features set is estimated using condition (8.8) and then a support value-based score is calculated using condition (8.9). Finally, the Euclidean distance between the training and testing score esteems is calculated to match the score. The data is recognized if the Euclidean distance assessment is less than the threshold; otherwise, the data is not recognized. Condition denotes value-based fusion support for the extracted features:

$$\tilde{S}_{value} = \left(c(f)+f(f)+i(f)\right) \Big/ c(f)*f(f)*i(f) \tag{8.8}$$

where $c(f)$ is the cavity-based feature, $f(f)$ is the filling-based feature, and $i(f)$ is the implant-based feature.

The score measure is depicted as, which is based on the support value, minimum and maximum value of all features.

$$S' = \tilde{S}_{value} + W_{\max} + W_{\min} \tag{8.9}$$

where

$$W_{\max} = \max\{all\ features\} \tag{8.10}$$

$$W_{\min} = \min\{all\ features\} \tag{8.11}$$

Matching Score

The Euclidean distance between the testing procedure score esteem and the training score esteem is calculated here. If the estimated distance is smaller than the threshold value, the implant is classed as a "cavity," "filling," or "implant":

$$\tilde{E}_D = \sqrt{\sum_{j=1}^{N}\left(S_{training}(j) - S_{testing}(j)\right)^2} \tag{8.12}$$

where $\tilde{E}_D$ is the Euclidean distance between training and testing score measures, $S_{training}$ is the score measure of the training set, and $S_{testing}$ is the score measure of the testing set. At last, the framework decides "cavity," "filling," and "implant" by the matching score.

8.4 Result and Discussion

The Python programming language is used to carry out the tasks mentioned. The accuracy, precision, recall, and F-measure are the performance parameters used to validate the models. In comparison to the existing systems AlexNet [14], CNN [15], and NASNet [16], the proposed model has a precision of 99.7%. The graph of performance measures is shown in Fig. 8.3. The suggested method's MAE, MSE, and RMSE value graphs are also plotted and compared to the existing aproaches. The algorithms for calculating performance metrics are shown in Table 8.1. Fig. 8.4 depicts the three classes of dentistry: cavity, filling, and implant.

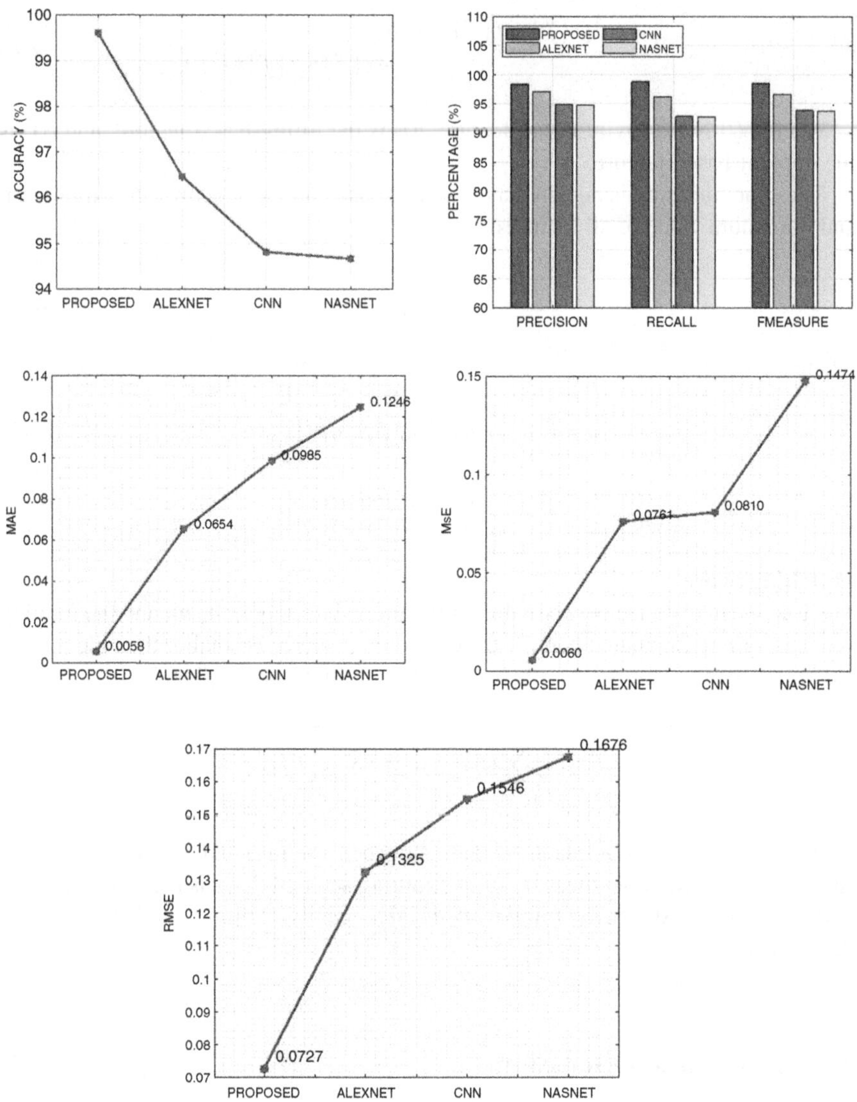

Fig. 8.3 Comparison of performance measures with the proposed and the existing methods

Figure 8.3 shows the graph of performance measures. The MAE, MSE, and RMSE value graphs are also plotted for the proposed and compared with the existing methods. Figure 8.3(a) shows the accuracy graph of comparison with the proposed existing methods AlexNet [14], CNN [15], and NASNet [16]. The accuracy reached is 99.7%, which is far better when compared with the existing methods, i.e., 96.4%, 94.4%, and 94.3%. Figure 8.3(b) shows the comparison of precision, recall, and F-measure proposed reaching 98% compared with the existing methods reaching low values. Figure 8.3(c) shows the MAE (mean absolute error) comparison

Table 8.1 Calculation formulae of the performance measures

Performance measures formula	
Accuracy	$\frac{(\mathrm{TN}+\mathrm{TP})}{(\mathrm{TN}+\mathrm{TP}+\mathrm{FN}+\mathrm{FP})}$
Precision	$\frac{TP}{TP+FP}$
Recall	$\frac{TP}{TP+FN}$
F-measure	$\frac{2TP}{2TP+FP+FN}$
RMSE (root mean square error)	$\sqrt{\frac{\sum_{x=1}^{N}\left(Z_x-\hat{Z}_x\right)^2}{N}}$
MAE (mean absolute error)	$\frac{\sum_{x=1}^{n}\lvert Q_x-P_x\rvert}{n}$
MSE (mean square error)	$\frac{1}{n}\sum_{x=1}^{n}\left(Z_x-\hat{Z}_x\right)^2$

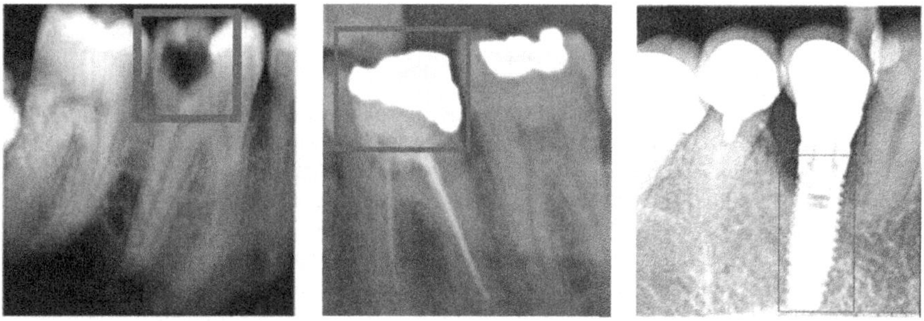

a) Cavity b) Filling c) Implant

Fig. 8.4 Classification of dentistry in three classes: cavity, filling, and implant

with the proposed existing methods AlexNet [14], CNN [15], and NASNet [16]. The MAE for the proposed system is as low as compared with the existing methods reaching high error rate. Figure 8.3(d) shows the MSE (mean square error) comparison with the proposed existing methods AlexNet [14], CNN [15], and NASNet [16]. The MSE for the proposed system is as low as compared with the existing methods reaching high error rate. Figure 8.3(e) shows the RMSE (root mean square error) comparison with the proposed existing methods AlexNet [14], CNN [15], and NASNet [16]. The RMSE for the proposed system is as low as compared with the existing methods reaching high error rate.

8.5 Conclusion

This research presents an x-ray image-based multiclass classification algorithm. The work used an entropy-based feature mapping approach to create a convolutional neural network. Fusion matching is based on support value classification. During the classification procedure, three different sorts of classes are used: cavity, filling, and implant. Multiple layers, dropout layers, and activation functions are used to apply image processing stages to neural networks. While the purpose of this research is to segment tooth instances, the technique shown here can be extended to other domains with similar issues, such as separating cell instances. When compared to existing approaches, better overcome were generated in this research.

References

1. Meier T, Deumelandt P, Christen O, Stangl GI, Riedel K, Langer M (2017) Global burden of sugar-related dental diseases in 168 countries and corresponding health care costs. J Dent Res 96:845–854
2. Pitts NB, Zero DT, Marsh PD, Ekstrand K, Weintraub JA, Ramos-Gomez F, Tagami J, Twetman S, Tsakos G, Ismail A (2017) Dental caries. Nat Rev Dis Primers 3:17030
3. James SL, Abate D, Abate KH, Abay SM, Abbafati C, Abbasi N, Abbastabar H, Abd-Allah F, Abdela J, Abdelalim A et al (2018) Global, regional, and national incidence, prevalence, and years lived with disability for 354 diseases and injuries for 195 countries and territories, 1990–2017: a systematic analysis for the global burden of disease study 2017. Lancet 392:1789–1858
4. Feng X (2018) Oral health status of Chinese residents: Report of the fourth oral health epidemiological survey in China. In: Proceedings of the 2018 18th annual meeting of oral preventive medicine of chinese stomatological association, Xi'an, China, p 2
5. Mathur VP, Dhillon JK (2018) Dental caries: a disease which needs attention. Indian J Pediatr 85:202–206
6. Lee J-H, Kim D-H, Jeong S-N, Choi S-H (2018) Detection and diagnosis of dental caries using a deep learning-based convolutional neural network algorithm. J Dent 77:106–111
7. Leo LM, Kalapalatha Reddy T (2021) Learning compact and discriminative hybrid neural network for dental caries classification. Microprocess Microsyst 82:103836
8. Tian S, Dai N, Zhang B, Yuan F, Qing Y, Cheng X (2019) Automatic classification and segmentation of teeth on 3D dental model using hierarchical deep learning networks. IEEE Access 7:84817–84828
9. Yauney G, Rana A, Wong LC, Javia P, Muftu A, Shah P (2019) Automated process incorporating machine learning segmentation and correlation of oral diseases with systemic health. In: *2019 41st annual international conference of the IEEE engineering in medicine and biology society (EMBC)*. IEEE, pp 3387–3393
10. Yöntemleri D, Güncel H, Tanı Ç (2016) Recent methods for diagnosis of dental caries in dentistry. Adnan Menderes University Faculty of Dentistry, Department of Pediatric Dentistry, Aydın, Turkey 1:29–36
11. Tuzoff DV, Tuzova LN, Bornstein MM, Krasnov AS, Kharchenko MA, Nikolenko SI, Sveshnikov MM, Bednenko GB (2019) Tooth detection and numbering in panoramic radiographs using convolutional neural networks. Dentomaxillofac Radiol 48(4):20180051
12. Zhang K, Ji W, Chen H, Lyu P (2018) An effective teeth recognition method using label tree with cascade network structure. Comput Med Imaging Graph 68:61–70

13. Xu X, Liu C, Zheng Y (2018) 3D tooth segmentation and labeling using deep convolutional neural networks. IEEE Trans Vis Comput Graph 25(7):2336–2348
14. AL-Ghamdi AS, Ragab M, AlGhamdi SA, Asseri AH, Mansour RF, Koundal D (2022) Detection of dental diseases through X-ray images using neural search architecture network. Comput Intell Neurosci 2022
15. Bhalla K, Koundal D, Bhatia S, Rahmani MKI, Tahir M (2022) Fusion of infrared and visible images using fuzzy based siamese convolutional network. Comput Mat Continua 70(3):5503–5518
16. Singh P, Kaur R (2020) An integrated fog and Artificial Intelligence smart health framework to predict and prevent COVID-19. Global Transit 2:283–292
17. Singh P, Kaur R (2021) Implementation of the QoS framework using fog computing to predict COVID-19 disease at early stage. World J Eng 19(1):80–89
18. Fukuda M (2020) Evaluation of an artificial intelligence system for detecting vertical root fracture on panoramic radiography. Oral Radiol 36(4):337–343
19. Zhang X, Liang Y, Li W, Liu C, Deao G, Sun W, Miao L (2022) Development and evaluation of deep learning for screening dental caries from oral photographs. Oral Dis 28(1):173–181
20. Kang I-A, Njimbouom SN, Lee K-O, Kim J-D (2022) DCP: prediction of dental caries using machine learning in personalized medicine. Appl Sci 12(6):3043
21. Reda R, Zanza A, Mazzoni A, Cicconetti A, Testarelli L, Di Nardo D (2021) An update of the possible applications of magnetic resonance imaging (MRI) in dentistry: a literature review. J Imag 7(5):75
22. Irfan M, Iftikhar MA, Yasin S, Draz U, Ali T, Hussain S, Bukhari S et al (2021) Role of hybrid deep neural networks (HDNNs), computed tomography, and chest X-rays for the detection of COVID-19. Int J Environ Res Public Health 18(6):3056

Index

K. Shaikh et al., *Artificial Intelligence in Dentistry*,
https://doi.org/10.1007/978-3-031-19715-4